CW00347915

ADVANCE PRAISE

'Hilarious, fascinating, and moving. A very special book about a very special family. I laughed and learned so much.'
Elis James

'There's so much love and good energy in this book. It had me smiling from the very first words.'
Adam Hills

'*Normal Schmormal* is a laugh-out-loud, touching memoir of advice, where embracing the weird becomes something wonderful. Every parent should have a copy.'
Emma Kennedy

'This is a must read. Ashley Blaker has a special brand of comic magic. His gift is in making the toughest life-challenges seem relatable and even joyous.'
Rob Rinder

'A very funny and honest account of Ashley's extraordinary ordinary life. There is treasure here for all parents, non-parents and children of parents, and that is surely most people.'
Alex Horne

'Funny and warm hearted, this book is a godsend for neurodivergent parents like me.'
Josie Long

'Absolutely hilarious and yet so poignant. This book is going to both entertain and bring comfort to so many people, giving them hope for the future.'
Matt Lucas

'Inspirational, moving and massively funny. A beautiful schmeautiful book.'
David Schneider

'Ashley is a superb comic writer and this is a brilliantly funny and often incredibly emotional memoir.'
David Walliams

'Full of love, this book is a unique and uplifting document of a remarkable everyday life. God knows how Ashley found time to write it.'
Mark Watson

'Funny, moving and incredibly useful. This book can teach us all something about parenting.'
Lucy Porter

'A vivid record of a father's love for his children and a plea for others to follow suit, whatever their kids may be like. A gorgeous book.'
Jeremy Dyson

'Chipped away at my ignorance and made me laugh at the same time. A neat trick.'
Mike Wozniak

'Great insights and advice for any parent, from a unique and fascinating family and their brilliantly funny dad.'
Katy Brand

ADVANCE CRITICISM

'Utter rubbish'
Adam Blaker

'Just lies to make us look bad'
Ollie Blaker

'The words are too bright for my ears'
Dylan Blaker

'If it sells a million copies,
how much LEGO will I get?'
Edward Blaker

'iPad not working'
Zoe Blaker

'Can I have a drink?'
Bailey Blaker

For Gemma, who does the real work.
I just wrote a book about it.

NORMAL SCHMORMAL

My occasionally helpful guide to parenting kids with special needs

ASHLEY BLAKER

HarperCollins*Publishers*

HarperCollins*Publishers*
1 London Bridge Street
London SE1 9GF

www.harpercollins.co.uk

HarperCollins*Publishers*
Macken House, 39/40 Mayor Street Upper
Dublin 1, D01 C9W8, Ireland

First published by HarperCollins*Publishers* 2023

1 3 5 7 9 10 8 6 4 2

A catalogue record of this book is
available from the British Library

ISBN 978-0-00-855811-6

Printed and bound in the UK using 100%
renewable electricity at CPI Group (UK) Ltd

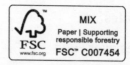

MIX
Paper | Supporting
responsible forestry
FSC
www.fsc.org
FSC™ C007454

This book is produced from independently certified FSC™ paper
to ensure responsible forest management.

For more information visit: www.harpercollins.co.uk/green

CONTENTS

ACKNOWLEDGEMENTS

There are many people to thank for their role in the creation of this book. First, thank you to my editor at HarperCollins, Anna Mrowiec, for her huge encouragement and expert guidance. It's been an absolute pleasure working with you and sharing several delicious lunches.

Thank you to my agent Vivienne Clore for her support, and also Cheryl Hayes, Carol Smith and everyone else at Vivienne Clore Management.

I owe an enormous debt of gratitude to Steve Doherty, who, as producer of my BBC Radio 4 show *Ashley Blaker: 6.5 Children*, has played a large role in the conception of this work. Without that series I would not have written this book. With that in mind, thank you to the Radio 4 controller Mohit Bakaya and the former commissioning editor of comedy Sioned Wiliam for their faith in me and interest in my family life. Thank you to the cast: Shelley Blond, Kieran Hodgson, Rosie Holt and Judith Jacob. Much appreciation too to my good friend Steve Hall for his many notes on the series, which have helped shape this book, and Gaby Jerrard for her PR work on the show.

Thank you to photographer extraordinaire Steve Ullathorne for his patience with my children as he tried to get them to pose for the cover photo. Even confronted with their usual Blaker belligerence, he still did a tremendous job.

Thank you to the friends who read parts of the book during the writing process and gave feedback, including Rhiannon Barber, Bonnie Carter, Hayley Dier, Erin Edmison, Matt Lucas, Ilana Ordman, Jennifer Schultz and Lauren Wilson. Big thanks to Stephanie Santiago who has followed this book from the very first word and given several great notes. Extra special thanks also to Megan Robinson for her constant support and cheerleading, especially at times when I was struggling to get going.

Thank you to the many professionals, charities and organisations who have been involved with our children, and extra special thanks to Kisharon School and KEF for their ongoing work with our eldest daughter. Likewise, our eternal gratitude to Laura and Ian Macmull for doing such an incredible job fostering her and for their continued friendship and support.

Thanks to my parents Philippa and Marshall Blaker for their involvement in the children's lives as precious grandparents, and for all they have done for both me and Gemma.

Of course, this book would not exist without my amazing children. Thank you to the six of them for being themselves in all their magnificent glory and providing so much material that the writing was relatively easy. I love each of you very much indeed.

Finally, my unending gratitude to Gemma, who has not only carried and given birth to five of these kids but has done all the hard work and been solely responsible for the wonderful people our children have become. I can only take ownership for their flaws. Thank you for all the selfless work you've done for me and our children.

LIST OF ABBREVIATIONS

ADD – Attention deficit disorder
ADHD – Attention deficit hyperactivity disorder
ASD – Autism spectrum disorder
AVSD – Atrioventricular septal defect
BEAM – Barnet Early Autism Model (basically an early
    intervention service run by our local council)
CAMHS – Child and adolescent mental health services
    (part of the NHS)
DS – Down syndrome (also the Nintendo of choice in
    our house until they brought out the Switch)
EHCP – Education, health and care plan
GOSH – Great Ormond Street Hospital
IEP – Individual education plan
LEA – Local education authority
LSA – Learning support assistant
NHS – National Health Service
OFSTED – The Office for Standards in Education,
    Children's Services and Skills. This is a
    non-ministerial department of government
    responsible for inspecting schools as well as many

other educational institutions. Consequently, the
mere mention of the word will cause many teachers
to metaphorically shit themselves. And most
headteachers to literally shit themselves.

PECS – Picture Exchange Communication System

SALT – Speech and language therapist

SEN – Special educational needs

SEND – Special educational needs and disabilities

SENDCo – Special educational needs and/or disabilities
  coordinator

SENDIST – Special Educational Needs and Disability
  Tribunal

SPD – Sensory processing disorder

SPLINK – (Find a) Safe place to stop, then cross; (stand
  on the) pavement near the curb; look all around for
  traffic; if traffic is coming, let it pass; (when there is)
  no traffic near, walk across the road; keep looking for
  traffic while you cross.

TEACCH – Teaching, Expanding, Appreciating,
  Collaborating and Cooperating with colleagues, and
  Holistic

PREFACE

Hello and welcome to my book. First of all, thank you very much for buying it. And if you haven't bought this copy and are just flipping through it in WHSmith to kill some time before a train or a flight, I wish you a lovely and safe trip. But only after taking this book to the till and purchasing it, if you don't mind.

If you hadn't already realised from the title, this book is about parenting children with special educational needs (or SEN, an abbreviation I'll often use to avoid repeating that term again and again, even though it would have helped me reach my word count more quickly). More importantly, though, this book is about *my* experience of parenting children with special educational needs. It's effectively a memoir, and although there are elements of how-to thrown in – and all being well, it will at least be *occasionally* helpful – it's certainly not intended to be a definitive guide. There are other works out there on this subject, and if that's what you're after, organisations like Mencap and the National Autistic Society have recommendations on their websites.

Obviously, you should still buy this book too, because I have some funny anecdotes that I hope you'll enjoy.

Among the reasons I have no intention of writing an out-and-out guide to having children with SEN is that there are lots of different kinds of needs, and I've had no first-hand involvement with most of them. Moreover, all children are different, so I don't want to make too many generalisations. Even if you also have children with autism, ADHD or Down syndrome, there will undoubtedly be stories in this book that will make you realise how much your kids are unlike mine. I'd imagine yours are better behaved for a start.

And come to think of it, all adults are different. So just because I've reacted one way to my children's diagnoses or their questionable social skills, it doesn't mean you'll have felt this way too. I can only speak for myself: a balding, out-of-shape man in his mid- to late 40s (depending on how generous you want to be with the word 'mid-'). I am also aware that while we have several children with varying levels of need, we still have it easier than most due to our many privileges. We're a white, middle-class, well-educated family, and although I always feel short of money, we aren't on the breadline, so it could definitely be a lot worse. We also benefit from living in a country with an NHS and state school system which, while both underfunded and frustratingly bureaucratic, means we have access to professionals who can give us much of the support that we need, all free of charge. Don't worry, we'll get round to those issues of red tape and their impact on us in due course.

Hopefully none of this is an issue because I'm not aiming to write mis-lit, or what's sometimes called 'misery porn', a term that always makes me imagine an adult video starring a Kathy Bates lookalike. You know, the kind of books that Waterstones place in a section called 'Painful Lives', which I feel could apply to me, but only because of my terrible athlete's foot and haemorrhoids. You'll be pleased to know I'm not here to depress you!* Quite the opposite, in fact, because I want to share some of the funnier sides to raising our children. Not surprising really, given that I'm a comedian. Finding the lighter side is what we do. And while there are many things I wish we hadn't had to go through, looking back I wouldn't swap our experiences for anything.

At risk of generalising, just a few hundred words after saying I don't want to generalise, I firmly believe there's great joy to be found in raising children with SEN. I've always thought the difference between conventional and SEN kids is akin to that between mainstream and more avant-garde musicians. Ordinary children are like Coldplay. A perfectly good band who are very popular, have some great songs and make lots of money. But let's be honest, Coldplay are a bit safe. There's nothing demanding about them; that's why they're so popular. Neither are they in any way cool.

Seeing myself as a bit of hipster muso in the John Peel mould – or possibly that Jazz Club character in *The Fast Show* – Coldplay were never the kind of music I wanted to listen to (or at least, not that I'd ever admit to in public).

---

* I say you'll be pleased to hear, but a quick Google search tells me that mis-lit has been called 'the book world's biggest boom sector', so it's quite possible that you'd prefer that this book were miserable, and for reasons of sales alone I should probably rethink before I write any further.

I was always drawn to the more experimental artists. Those that really challenged the listener, that didn't give a shit about pleasing the audience and were only interested in following their muse. You wouldn't see Frank Zappa or Captain Beefheart on the shelves in Tesco. They had far too much integrity to worry about fitting in with the mainstream. The musicians I like are rebellious, alternative, and yes, cool.

Frank Zappa, Captain Beefheart, Patti Smith, even Björk: they are the SEN children. Yes, of course it would be simpler to have mainstream children, in much the same way that it would be easier to sit in the car and put on *Parachutes*. But I've never been one to head down the easy route like everyone else. And so, just as I'd rather drive to Beefheart's *Trout Mask Replica* or Kate Bush's *The Dreaming*, I personally love the fact I have kids with special needs. They possess the same 'don't give a fuck' attitude as Zappa and Beefheart, are too cool for (mainstream) school and are only interested in doing things their way rather than following the herd. And in both cases, I can walk around with a wonderful sense of superiority. I don't listen to the music that most people listen to, nor am I raising the kids that most people are raising. They aren't for hipsters like us. We, and all the other parents of SEN kids, are connoisseurs, doing the *real* parenting that would probably be a bit too challenging for everyone else. Mmmmm, nice!

As for the format of the book, I wanted to tell you about my experiences with our children but didn't want to get too bogged down with all the chronology. I was also keen to make it as accessible as possible, with headings that were potentially useful to other parents in our situation. That is why I've opted for an A to Z, though fittingly for a book about children who often find learning difficult and who refuse to follow the normal rules, the letters are jumbled up in a seemingly random order. If you find this incredibly frustrating, then welcome to my life.

Speaking of frustration, I wanted to affirm right at the top that while I find much of my children's behaviour infuriating, I love them all exactly as they are. I'll probably restate this numerous times in the book, but my editor insisted I declare it now in case any reader should doubt just how important my kids are to me. Plus, my children demanded I proclaim it immediately, presumably because they weren't entirely convinced themselves. Sorry, Blakers, I do love you very much!

We're nearly ready to dive in, so I sincerely hope you enjoy reading this book and get something out of it. I wish to apologise in advance for any crappy dad jokes, though in fairness, being a father to six, I feel I should be permitted more than the usual quota. If you too are the parent of a *Zappa*, you'll doubtless recognise much of what I'm writing about, and will nod along to our similar experiences. And if you're the mum or dad to a *Coldplay*, or if you're not a parent at all, I would love you to learn something about our lives so perhaps you can empathise with those who have children like mine. Because although this is my story, it is ultimately an account of being an SEN parent. I view this book as being for all of us: to be seen, to say our piece, so the world knows what our lives look like. I dedicate this book to you all (although the royalties will stay solely with me, I'm afraid). Don't worry about what's normal. Normal schmormal. Just keep doing what you're doing and hopefully with a smile on your face.

With much love
Ashley

INTRODUCTION

Before we get going with my promised 'occasionally helpful guide to parenting kids with special needs', let me introduce the players in my story and tell you a little bit about how we got here. Don't worry, I'll keep it brief and then fill in the blanks as we go.

I'm **Ashley**. That much you should be aware of by now, seeing as you're holding my book. I'm the father of six children, or what I call a Blaker's half-dozen.* I work as a stand-up comedian and live in north London, apart from when I'm performing on tour, when I manage to dodge some of my parental duties. Getting out of our lengthy bedtime routine is probably the only upside to a night in a Travelodge.

Prior to having kids, I'd had some experience of people with learning difficulties. At school we had an annual Mencap Funday, when local children and young adults, many with Down syndrome, would come for a day of activities. This prompted me to volunteer for two years

---

* I did warn you about the dad jokes.

every Wednesday evening at the Mencap Jubilee Club in Borehamwood. But while I took great pleasure from this experience, I can't say it really prepared me for what was to come. My understanding of autism was mostly taken from *Rain Man* – we'll deal with that film and its faults a bit later – and I didn't know any of the countless abbreviations with which I'm now familiar. As you'll soon discover, the world of SEN parenting is absolutely full of abbreviations. Starting, of course, with SEN.*

I want to acknowledge immediately that the poor woman doing most of the work in our house is the children's mother, my wife **Gemma**. She is currently a Year One teacher and the Head of Teaching and Learning in a local primary school. She is also the Head of Teaching and Learning in our house, although I'd say she is much more successful in her paid job than she is in this unpaid one, especially if the pupils are meant to learn about brushing their teeth and washing up their dirty plates. She had previously been a stay-at-home mum for ten years, as necessitated by the quite ridiculous number of appointments our children seem to have. Prior to that, I'd been the stay-at-home parent, as required not only by the appointments, but demanded by the London Borough of Hackney when we adopted a daughter in 2010.

Before stopping work for a decade, Gemma had been a SENDCo (special educational needs and/or disabilities coordinator) at two different secondary schools, and then a headteacher at a special school. She was handily picking up much useful experience ahead of us effec-

---

* I'll explain most of them as we go, but there's also a handy list of abbreviations at the front of the book.

tively running our own special school right here in our home. Because not only do we have a very full life with half a dozen kids, we also have several other major challenges. And that's before we get to my ICU-level athlete's foot and piles.

I'm not totally sure why we started having children so quickly and in such high volume. I seem to remember suggesting that we should take our relationship to the next level by adding an extra person. Unfortunately, Gemma misunderstood my hints and thought this meant starting a family. Consequently, having been married merely a few months, we began trying to produce a child. I had only just produced *Little Britain* for Radio 4, but Gemma and I would soon be creating characters every bit as outlandish as Matt Lucas and David Walliams's, and somehow with even more vomiting. Sadly, when it comes to catchphrases, 'Yeah but no but yeah but no' proved a lot more marketable than 'I need £10' and 'It's my turn on the Xbox.'

Before I tell you about the children, I want to stress that they are very much more than their diagnoses. I am going to list them here merely so you can begin to get some idea of what our lives look like on a daily basis. So, starting with those with a recognised need:

Adam is my eldest son and, as I write this, he's coming up to his 18th birthday. He was diagnosed with autism and ADHD (attention deficit hyperactivity disorder) as a three-year-old, which was prompted by his severe speech delay and incredibly limited diet. He's now growing into a wonderful young man, who, while a little shy, can be personable, responsible and easy-going. In fact, I'd guess that if you met him, you wouldn't even realise he was autistic because through a combination of maturity, medication and self-taught coping mechanisms (possibly including what is sometimes called 'masking'), he presents as if he were any other teenage boy.

However, it wasn't always thus. At varying stages Adam has been an almost entirely non-verbal toddler who attended a specialist nursery provision; a wild force of nature who terrified anyone and everyone with whom he came into contact; and a cunning presence in our house, forever plotting how any circumstance could be controlled to serve his needs. Adam was so expert at manipulating every situation to benefit his own desires that he could have authored Machiavelli's *The Prince*, were it written by someone who failed GCSE English. This is mostly due to his diagnosis, but I imagine can also be put down to pure Blaker belligerence.

Dylan is my third son and is currently 14 years old. He was diagnosed with autism and ADHD at age six. Having been through this once with Adam, we were primed to spot the signs, although as clues go, not being able to talk at six years old wouldn't have got past even Scooby Doo and Shaggy. Dylan now attends a mainstream state secondary school and, like Adam, he comes across like any other long-haired, messy and phenomenally cantankerous boy of his age. He is also very talented at art, and last year was chosen as one of the contestants on the BBC series *Britain's Best Young Artist*. Dylan's experience on this show actually brought home to us some of the ways in which his autism affects him, but again, were you to have seen Dylan on TV or if you met him in the street, you'd not immediately realise this was someone with any kind of additional need at all.

As with Adam, this apparent normality is a relatively new development. Previously, Dylan existed predominantly in his own self-contained bubble of strangeness from which he departed less frequently than package holidays to the Wuhan wet markets. Having not spoken for six years, he appeared determined to make up for lost time. At any given moment he could launch into a half-hour soliloquy of gibberish in a monotone voice that was perfectly pitched to send people to sleep. Not ideal when you're driving, but amazing when you have a baby in the car who'd benefit from an afternoon nap. Even now, ask Dylan how his day went and don't be surprised if he answers with a monologue about whether Batman is a human who's a bat or a bat who's a human or if he's a human and a bat at the same time because he saw a film online that said humans are more closely related to bats than they are apes. We have often wondered what part of this is the result of his autism and what is just the effect of watching too many videos on YouTube and TikTok.

The final child diagnosed with special educational needs is our adopted daughter **Zoe**, who has Down syndrome (or DS, an abbreviation that I'll use in this book but never at home since it would suggest the children's old Nintendo devices. If I told any of my sons that Zoe had DS they'd be freaking out with anger, even though they've long since upgraded to the Nintendo Switch). She is now 13 and has lived with us since she was two and a half years old. Therefore, she is the fourth oldest but was the fifth to come along. And if that sounds confusing, be warned, you've not even heard the half of it yet. The full tale of her adoption is to follow, but for now a brief summary of life with Zoe.

Well, in many ways she's by far and away the most impressive member of the Blaker household, probably due in no small part to the fact she isn't biologically mine. She isn't manipulative, doesn't talk endless rubbish and has almost none of the further terrible habits of our other children. On the contrary, she has a generally sunny nature and would charm even the most hard-hearted of people with her beautiful smile. Those that meet Zoe or work with her, whether at school or Sunday club, instantly fall in love with her.

Of course, these people don't get the full Zoe experience, because spending a few hours with someone isn't the same as living with them. If they did, they'd know Zoe can be as challenging as any of our children. Like many with DS, alongside her learning difficulties she's had issues with her heart, mobility, muscle tone, hearing, sight and stomach. The day she moved into our house my calendar immediately filled up with regular appointments to visit every possible kind of specialist. Meanwhile my car practically learnt how to drive itself to Great Ormond Street Hospital.* And crucially, while Adam and Dylan's autism has become less noticeable as they've aged, Zoe has become more demanding. We are now trying to parent a child with the mental age of a four-year-old, but who is also going through puberty, and has all the usual hormones starting to race through her body.

Those are our children – the first, third and fourth or fifth, depending on how you look at it – that have official diagnoses given to them by NHS professionals. Our other

---

* Or GOSH, for fans of all the abbreviations.

children merely have labels bestowed on them by me and Gemma, not least of which is the surname Blaker, pretty much a diagnosis on its own.

Our second son, **Ollie**, is approaching 17 but thinks of himself as closer to 25. If you met him, you'd probably imagine this too. He attends school, when he can be bothered to turn up, but also works part-time in a local supermarket. In many ways this has been great for him, but putting money in his pocket and surrounding him with older colleagues has also given him a touch too much arrogance. The word 'insouciance' could have been invented for Ollie. He's notorious among his peers for walking into lessons half an hour late, usually with a bacon sandwich from Greggs in his hand. That would be excessively nonchalant in any school, but in a Jewish institution it's really taking the piss.

Being just 13 months younger than Adam, Ollie is unsurprisingly very close to his older brother. They have been inseparable for most of the past 16-plus years, sharing a room for much of that time, and have developed a somewhat symbiotic relationship. Ollie has veered between looking up to Adam, and being his carer and translator, their partnership reaching its apogee at primary school, when they formed a business selling sweets in the playground. In this junior version of Trotters Independent Traders, Ollie was the brains of the operation. He would work out the profit margins and strategise how to beat the competition, with Adam sent out as the nominal shopkeeper. Unfortunately, the headteacher caught them and put the firm into receivership before we could find out whether by the same time next year they'd be millionaires.

Ollie is now back selling sweets, among other groceries, and while everyone who shops in the supermarket tells me he's such a wonderfully polite boy, he seems to reserve this for the customers. When at home he appears to be constantly furious with the entire world, and will scream and swear at anyone who dares interact with him. Although living in this house, I can't say I blame him.

Official diagnosis: nothing. Regular *Coldplay*.

My personal diagnosis: anger issues and staggering insolence. Or, put more concisely, a teenager.

Our fourth son is **Edward**, who is 12 years old. He isn't angry at all and is the most sanguine, lovely boy, in many ways the least challenging of all our children. However, he is definitely no *Coldplay*, even if he doesn't have any paperwork to prove it. For a start, he was born with a hole in his heart, which he had closed by surgery when he was six years old. As a result of his cardiac issues, he is much smaller than everyone else his age, although this only adds to his inherent cuteness. He may grow in time, but these heart concerns will be with him for life. We received a letter only this past week saying that because of his heart surgery, he must never get any piercings or tattoos. I am of course devastated that he won't ever be able to prove his loyalty to our football team by having a liver bird inked on his body.

Beyond the physical issues, there are more telling signs that Edward isn't just any old *Coldplay*. I'd even go so far as to say he exhibits more classic signs of autism than any of the others. Many children with ASD (we've not had an abbreviation for quite a few paragraphs, so here's another one for you – autism spectrum disorder) enjoy lining up their toys and display hyperfixation: the complete immersion in something to the exclusion of everything else. Well, for as long as I can remember, Edward has done nothing but rearrange identical bits of LEGO on a shelf, all of which have a meaning that only he can decipher. He does this while continually watching and rewatching the *Star Wars* saga, to the point I'm not sure if he has a better relationship with me or Yoda. Hmmm, normal this is not.

The obvious question is why he doesn't have a diagnosis, and the simple answer is that nothing has prompted us to seriously investigate it. Once, in a meeting with Adam's psychiatrist at our local CAMHS (Child and Adolescent Mental Health Services), Gemma did raise Edward's name and described his behaviour. The doctor responded that he would be happy to assess him, but that frankly no one would ever believe that we had a fourth child with special needs, and so it was probably best to keep it to ourselves! We already had our hands full with the three *Zappas*, and Edward has never had any learning difficulty that would have benefited from getting him evaluated for an IEP (individual education plan) or EHCP (education, health and care plan). He is just a little boy who is excessively obsessed with LEGO. And *Star Wars*. And Marvel movies. Oh, and dinosaurs.

Official diagnosis: nothing. Regular *Coldplay*.

My personal diagnosis: are you serious?! I have just laid out more clues than Miss Marple does immediately before she names the murderer.

Our sixth and final child, whichever way you calculate it, is our daughter **Bailey**, who makes the other five look easy. She is an eight-year-old but, like Ollie, she doesn't seem to believe it. Five years ago she was already a threenager. These days she's more like a university fresher trapped in the body of a Year Three pupil. Her main interests are clothes, make-up and pouting in selfies, and she calls everyone, including both her parents, 'girlfriend'. Even more irritatingly, she's started referring to herself not only in the third person – that would be bad enough – but preceded by the definite article. She doesn't say, 'Those crisps belong to me'; she says, 'Those crisps belong to The Bailey.' I don't know which American show she's been watching, but I want to kill whoever wrote it!

The other thing everyone notices about Bailey – and I really do mean everyone who has spent at least a couple of minutes with her – is that she simply never shuts up. For those for whom it is literally a couple of minutes, this is rather adorable. They love hearing about what The Bailey has been learning in school, what she's been doing at Brownies, her favourite YouTube channels and what make-up she'd like to buy, girlfriend. For those of us that live with her, it's bordering on torture. Bailey is going to tell us her news no matter what, and she won't be deterred by us working, sleeping, using the toilet or even being deep in conversation with someone else.

I have often wondered if the universe is just taking the piss out of us with Bailey. That after several sons with severe speech delay, we've now been given a child that is too far in the opposite direction. We never had to wait for Bailey to start talking. She began at the appropriate age and has barely paused for breath ever since. The only time she ever stops is to show us one of the energetic dance routines she's devised – typically to a song from

The Greatest Showman or *Six* – or to perform one of her own self-penned numbers such as the unforgettable 'Smelly Poopy, Yeah'. I would share the lyrics with you, but you've just seen them. It's 'Smelly poopy, yeah' repeated ad infinitum. Nonetheless, I've no doubt her *joie de vivre* and natural charisma will get her far because she charms everyone she meets, from other children at school to checkout staff in shops.

According to the NHS website, excessive talking and interrupting conversations are among the main signs of ADHD, as are hyperactivity and disproportionate physical movement. However, I'm still not convinced these traits mark her out as anything more than a *Coldplay* with lots to get off her chest. Bailey's monologues – is it even called a monologue if it never has a clear start and end point?! – aren't the bizarre stream of consciousness that Dylan specialises in. You're not going to hear Bailey ruminate on whether she'd rather live in the Arctic or Antarctic, which in fairness was probably one of Dylan's less unusual soliloquies. She sticks to factual things like the events of her day, just recited in excruciating detail. 'And then I said to Katie ... and then she was like ... and then I was like ... and then she was like ... and then I was like ...' and so on and so on.

And if I'm looking for small mercies, at least Bailey doesn't use Dylan's monotone delivery. On the contrary, she displays a remarkable range of emotions for an eight-year-old. Excitement. Over-excitement. Feverish excitement. Delirious excitement. Please, for the love of God, just stop talking about make-up for two minutes excitement. And just as we decided not to get Edward assessed, the same reasons apply to Bailey. She isn't doing too badly academically, so in truth I'm not sure help is required here. Ear plugs, yes, but an LSA (learning support assistant), probably not. And while I remain convinced no one should have this much to say for themselves, we've already got our hands sufficiently full to start contemplating any more meetings with specialists.

Official diagnosis: nothing. Regular *Coldplay*.

My personal diagnosis: well, she's got something, surely?! Sadly, one thing she doesn't have is an off button.

So that's the final reckoning. A score draw. Three *Zappas* to three *Coldplays*. And unless any of the latter group gets an official diagnosis, this is how it will remain, because one thing that's for sure is that we aren't adding to our children. When Bailey – sorry, The Bailey – was born in January 2014, Gemma told me in no uncertain terms that that shop was now closed. She was clearly ahead of her time, because this was a full six years before every other shop closed, and in this case there was no offer of a take-over from Asos.

Given all the above, perhaps the shop should have shut a little earlier. Some would argue that two boys with autism, or maybe even one, would have been enough work, and they'd have a point. The trouble is, unlike with other disabilities, ASD is not evident at birth. Midwives don't look at parents and say, 'Your child is neurodiverse.' ASD is something that becomes apparent with the passage of time and is then assessed by professionals. In Adam's case he was diagnosed after three years; with Dylan it took six. Therefore, even though our eldest son barely slept for the first year, didn't feed properly and cried almost non-stop from colic, we willingly decided to have another child only a few months later. In fact, Adam was still undiagnosed when we concluded that having a two-year-old and a one-year-old wasn't quite enough work, and started trying for a third. I think we'd just gone full-on Del Boy and decided sleep is for wimps. Had we known the extent of Adam's needs, then perhaps we'd have quit while we were behind. Instead, in our blissful ignorance, we ploughed on.

To some extent this lack of knowledge was to our benefit. In 2010, when we began the process of adopting Zoe, we believed we were the parents of just one autistic son. More importantly, the London Borough of Hackney believed we were the parents of just one autistic son. Indeed, our experience with having a child with SEN was one of the reasons they thought we could be suitable adopters of a girl with Down syndrome. However, if our then three-year-old Dylan had been diagnosed at this point, I'm sure Hackney would have said we had far too much on our plate to be considered. Possibly we'd have thought the same, although even the least astute reader will have already realised that if nothing else we are gluttons for punishment. Our bravery/stupidity is such that I imagine nothing would have stopped us trying to adopt Zoe, but obviously we'll never know. Unaware of what extra needs we had in our midst, on we went.

And as challenging as it all is, I'd not have it any different. We love our children just the way they are (and this time my editor didn't prompt me to say this). We love them as they are despite the endless meetings, assessments, therapists, public humiliations, failed playdates, soiled nappies, occasional violence, horrific hygiene, relentless quotations from *Star Wars*, Machiavellian plotting that would make a Bond villain blush, and surreal monologues about whether 'trees are more intelligent than humans because I saw a video on YouTube that said trees actually had a brain and that if the planet exists long enough then trees may evolve until they can do jobs'. I need to work so hard to entertain an audience, but I can make Zoe laugh like a drain simply by squeezing her hand or going, 'Daddy, say Daddy.' And it's not just sweet, innocent Zoe. My autistic boys bring me great pleasure too, even though they can't always do what a *Coldplay* can. And if you want to know what the challenges and rewards are of raising our special children, then please read on. My A–Z begins with …

1

M IS FOR MEETINGS, MEETINGS, MEETINGS

When I look at the lives of the parents of nearly all *Coldplays*, one of the things I envy most is their time. Now that's not to say raising a *Coldplay* won't involve all manner of chores that will inevitably fill your day. Many mums and dads will happily (or more accurately, unhappily) moan to you about having to do the school run followed by weeknights and weekends ferrying their offspring to playdates, birthday parties, music lessons, sports practice, swimming, martial arts and whichever gendered branch of Lord Baden-Powell's movement they deem most suitable. Of course, the shrewd parent will simply opt for drama club, where their precocious child can learn how to improvise all the other activities in their bedroom, while they relax downstairs with a glass of wine.

Yet my sympathy is very limited when it comes to any complaints of this kind. First, much of this is self-inflicted. Yes, children are required to go to school, and birthday parties are perhaps an annoying side-effect of having kids with friends. However, thereafter it's only middle-class paranoia and attempting to keep up with the other Tiger Mums that demands your little one attend ballet, drumming and Cantonese lessons. Will it really help them in later life? I personally spent my entire childhood refusing to take part in anything that involved me leaving the house and was the only boy at primary school who didn't go to judo or Cubs, staying home to watch *Grange Hill* instead. My parents weren't happy about my inactivity and worried I was missing out, but looking back I saved them hours in the car ferrying me around and I've never felt disadvantaged in my inability to tie a perfect Alpine Butterfly Loop. On the contrary, I was better off than my classmates because I got to watch Zammo's descent into heroin addiction and was able to digest the takeaway message to 'Just Say No'.*

Second, even if all these extra-curricular activities lead to busy evenings and weekends, at least the parents of *Coldplays* have the bulk of their weekdays free to get some work done. Sadly, like all parents of children with SEN, our lives involve a never-ending succession of meetings with professionals, all of which are slap bang in the middle of the day, presumably because these professionals have their own children who in the evening need to be taken to Cantonese lessons. How very inconsiderate of them.

Putting all the hospital appointments to one side (see 'X is for X-rays and Other Hospital Appointments' for

---

* I should clarify that to the best of my knowledge none of my peers became drug addicts either. Perhaps their parents videoed *Grange Hill* for them to watch later.

more on that), something parents of *Coldplays* will be blissfully unaware of is how much time we spend attending meetings at our children's schools. And why would they realise? If you don't include the daily school run – at which point most will be as swift as possible, so they don't have to hear how Naomi is now Grade 4 at oboe and Samuel is fluent in Mandarin (he already mastered Cantonese last year) – they might only visit twice a year for parents' evening. Even this may be a thing of the past since the COVID-enforced Zoom parents' evening is sure to be one of those innovations that remains post-pandemic. It works for everyone: parents don't have to leave the house, and teachers can be stricter with the over-chatty mums and dads by booting them out of the meeting room the second they've outstayed their welcome.

In contrast, most of our occasional time free from hospital appointments is taken up with school meetings. I've had days where there's been so much driving back and forth, I've been tempted to ask if I'd be allowed to stay and join the Reception class. At the very least, I would get a free lunch and it's got to be more nutritious than anything I'd normally feed myself. During the past 15 years I think we've attended every possible kind of school meeting:

Assessment meeting
Review meeting
Planning meeting
Pre-planning meeting
Beginning of term meeting
Middle of term meeting

End of term meeting
Transition between terms meeting
Emergency meeting
In case of emergency meeting
What can be learnt after the emergency despite all
    the planning meetings meeting

And those are just the standard meetings that are to be expected as parents of a *Zappa*. There are also those surprise ones that will inevitably pop up during the year, almost always at the most inconvenient time possible. We've had Adam's *Learning support assistant will be off for an afternoon next week pre-planning meeting*; Dylan's *Change of desk transition meeting*; and, most memorably, Zoe's *Which brand of batteries should go in her hearing aid planning meeting*. In case you wondered, after an hour of arguing we got our way and her school reluctantly agreed to opt for Duracell ahead of Energizer. Then a week later we were told that this size of battery isn't made by Duracell. We graciously accepted the school's apology for wasting yet more of our time, but turned down their invitation to attend an *Explanation as to why we didn't realise what companies make batteries for Zoe's hearing aid emergency meeting*. You must draw the line somewhere.

I'm still not quite sure why schools are so desperate to drag us in at every opportunity. Raising a kid with SEN is already challenging enough, so why make our lives even harder, forcing us to fill our precious child-free time by discussing the children in their absence? One would hope that their teachers – people with actual first-hand experience of how demanding our children can be – would have a little sympathy and cut us some slack. If they don't appreciate our plight, then no one will. Moreover, most teachers are themselves mums and dads, so they should be aware of the value of time away from one's offspring. Whether you're the parent of a *Coldplay* or a *Zappa*, if you have any period without a child in the house, then it's imperative you use it wisely. That will mean different things to different people: doing paid work, completing household chores, taking a nap, shopping, having sex, watching *Loose Women*. (Out of interest, I've just described my perfect day.) No one would think that heading back to their child's school to have yet another meeting is a good use of their time, unless it was a particularly crap episode of *Loose Women* that afternoon.

I thought we had an arrangement that we'd do the childcare in turns. I know it's never been discussed publicly, but surely it's an unspoken agreement. The Teacher–Parent Treaty of 1874. That we'd concentrate on mornings, evenings and weekends; and they'd do 8 a.m. until 4 p.m. Mondays to Fridays. Trust me, we're getting the short end of the stick here. Not only are the teachers paid while we're doing this gratis, they're also avoiding the nightmare that is the morning routine. And the nightmare that is the bedtime routine. Plus, they get 13 weeks off in addition to bank holidays. Those are never much fun for parents. The more I think about it, this is sounding like a pretty shitty arrangement to me. So, teachers, please don't make it even worse by bringing us into school on your shift. We don't make you come to our home to help give Zoe her bath in the evening. Why can't you just be grateful that you've got by far the better side of the deal and leave it at that before anyone tries to renegotiate this frankly unfair arrangement?

I am sure the reason for the endless meetings, like so many things that happen in schools nowadays, is simply bureaucracy. It seems that teachers being left alone to teach has gone the same way as schoolmasters employing the cane, smoking a pipe in front of the children, or inviting pupils onto his boat and encouraging them to touch his penis. Or was that just my school where this happened?*

The job of teaching has changed immeasurably in the last two decades, and local authorities and OFSTED (oh, come on, I know it's an abbreviation, but just google it if you really need to know what it stands for!) now have teachers tearing their hair out due to their insistence on all manner of protocols, red tape and form-filling. Every school requires a policy for everything from Healthy Eating to Whistleblowing, which is obviously a policy about making complaints, not which teacher is allowed to blow the whistle at the end of breaktime. Although if you told me there was a policy for that too, I wouldn't be all that surprised.

It's in the context of this love for process and paper trails that us parents end up enduring countless visits to schools, to sit in countless meetings about, in our case, our almost countless SEN children. And while I have sympathy for teachers who probably want to be there no more than we do, I feel we're the ones that are really

---

* In fairness, terrible things like this still happen in schools, but these days it will end up with teachers going to prison rather than being discreetly asked to find somewhere else to teach.

suffering here. They're not only doing their jobs, but they're also managing a brief escape from the classroom and getting some adult company for a change. I, on the other hand, can't ever get anything done because I'm so often called in for these meetings. I've already had to leave the house twice during the writing of this chapter, first for a *Zoe's period is coming sooner or later emergency meeting*, and then for the children's collective *Therapy for the after-effects of being discussed in hardback pre-planning meeting*. Don't worry, I'm sure they'll schedule similar meetings for both the audiobook and paperback. If you think this book isn't quite as good as you'd hoped it would be, then no wonder considering I keep having to stop what I'm doing to go to school, all in order to talk about something that could just as easily have been dealt with in a five-minute phone call.

In fact, any minor suspense about how the meeting will go is usually short-lived. Not because I am convinced any interaction with school will always be negative. Believe it or not, we've had some encouraging meetings as well. Not often, obviously, but they have happened. No, the reason for the lack of doubt is because experience tells me that everything can be gleaned from a quick glance at the table. Are there biscuits laid out? If so, great. This is going to be a positive one. In our case, that means our child has remarkably done something vaguely in line with their chronological age, give or take a few years. However, if you go into the meeting room and instead of a plate of biscuits there's a box of tissues, this isn't going to go well.

I'm so used to this that I've been to school meetings, spotted the tissues, and immediately claimed I needed to go home to switch off the oven. Then I've turned my phone off for the rest of the day and hoped by the time the school finally catches up with me, my child will have done something biscuit-worthy. It's not because I don't want to hear bad news about my child. That I'm used to by now. It's more because a box of tissues at a meeting can only mean one thing: we're going to need more meetings. My sons are keeping Kleenex in business, and while I'm aware most parents of teenage boys would say this, mine have boosted tissue sales pretty much since birth.

We've had so many of these meetings over the years that no matter what the occasion, any sighting of tissues is now a total trigger for Gemma. Just a brief glimpse of a travel packet in Sainsbury's is enough to provoke uncontrollable crying. One minor positive of the empty shelves at the start of the pandemic was that we could finally return to the supermarket without fear of seeing reminders of the *Tissues of Doom*. Gemma is adamant the tissues are only ever provided by male teachers, who seem to think offering them proves that they are sensitive and caring without having to properly respond to any of your issues. The upshot is, for Gemma, not only are the tissues a portent of more meetings, but they have also come to represent thousands of years of patriarchy.

Probably my least favourite of all the meetings – yes, even worse than 2013's classic *How to stop Dylan eating the textbooks emergency meeting* – is the annual *Transition meeting*. For those who aren't in the know, this is held towards the end of the academic year, to plan for – wait for it – a transition of some manner. The clues were in the title. Sometimes this could precede a big change, such as from primary to secondary school, but more commonly concerns the move from one year to the next.

There are several reasons I hate this one, even though it technically falls into the plate of biscuits category. First, the number of people present can feel overwhelmingly large. Attending a *Teaching Adam that swearing isn't big or clever planning meeting* might have been humiliating, but at least it only involved Adam's teacher and LSA. I'll never forget us seriously debating whether 'wanger' technically qualified as a swearword, an episode forever remembered in our family as 'Wangergate'.* The *Transition meeting*, on the other hand, can comprise so many people, the chance of getting your hands on the good biscuits is next to zero. I'm only interested in the custard creams, party rings and jammy dodgers. Once we're down to the stale digestives I think I'd rather have the box of tissues, if only to spit the biscuits into.

This is the granddaddy of all school meetings, so you'll get the parents, obviously, the current teacher, next year's teacher, the current LSA, next year's LSA if the current LSA is moving on because they're sick of being called a 'wanger', the SENDCo, and in some cases we've even had the headteacher showing up. Ostensibly this was to ensure the meeting went smoothly but was more likely due to the fact he wanted the Cadbury's Fingers. Even notwithstanding the fight over the food, seeing this many people can be intimidating, especially when everyone else knows each other and are colleagues. We're the outsiders coming in, and while they usually try to be nice, there's always a feeling that

---

* Upshot: it didn't, but they'd still rather he stopped saying it.

private conversations have already taken place in the staffroom.

Another reason I so dislike the *Transition meeting* is the way the current teacher must try to hide their relief that they are finally getting rid of our son. To their credit, they make an effort, but it's normally apparent on their face: a look that can only be described as demob happy. Even worse is the way they endeavour to keep things positive: remember, this is a plate of biscuits meeting. So, they cobble together a list of all our son's dubious achieve-ments – 'He's not chewed any books for a month'; 'On the school trip he only called five people a wanger' – and then avoid saying anything too negative. They're clearly in a rush to get us out the room so they can tell each other what's truly going on, and no doubt break out the real biscuits.

Personally, I find their use of euphemisms even worse than if they just came out with their honest opinion. Adam would be called a 'rather lively boy', which trans-lated means 'absolutely uncontrollable'. In the same vein, Dylan has been described as 'very much his own person', meaning 'completely in his own world and we have no idea what the hell's going on in his head'. Worst of all is seeing the look of utter horror on the face of next year's teacher. They're not going to be fooled by any of the polite terms used to spare our embarrassment. They speak the lingo and usually aren't sufficiently poker-faced to hide their fear of what's to come. Pah! You're scared? We have to *live* with these kids!

We've also had the misfortune of attending some particularly fraught meetings that were not only in the box of tissues category, but disproved Gemma's point about the patriarchy, since I don't think anyone – male or female – had the slightest desire to show themselves as sensitive and caring. Probably the worst was at Adam's primary school when they called us in to explain why they didn't want him to take part in the end of Year Six residential trip.

A brief prelude: this annual outing, at the very end of the children's time at primary school, was the culmination of eight years together and a rite of passage. The children had been talking about little else for months, and the parents' WhatsApp group was likewise preoccupied with discussion of this five-day trip to Cornwall. So, unsurprisingly, it was a crushing blow to be told that Adam wasn't welcome.

I can still picture the teachers' faces as they shifted uneasily in their seats and avoided our eyes, instead looking at each other in the hope of back-up. It's vaguely possible that they gave us a rational explanation as to why Adam couldn't attend. I think I was in shock seeing that they delivered the news almost immediately, with practically no small talk. But if this was the case, then the bombshell clearly afflicted Gemma too, because neither of us have the slightest recollection of anything approaching a coherent argument. Our joint memory is of the Year Six teacher, SENDCo and headteacher each stumbling over their words as they blamed a shortage of staff – they didn't have anyone to be with Adam for the duration of the trip – and the fact that our son wouldn't, in their humble opinion, be able to cope with the change of environment. They wanted him to come, that went without saying – although they'd say it again and again to stress the point – but sadly, it just wasn't possible.

The tension in the room was palpable, and things became more heated during the following half-hour. At one point I suggested that I join the trip, which would answer their supposed issue about lack of staffing. This was batted away with the claim that there were already too many parents coming along, and I should have signed up when they first asked for mums and dads willing to help. Yes, clearly it was my fault for not having the clairvoyance to know that in two weeks they'd say Adam couldn't attend without support, so I'd better volunteer now.

At one point Gemma mentioned very calmly that this was actually illegal, seeing as the school was required to make reasonable adjustments to accommodate Adam and any other children with SEN. This was met with a completely not-calm response from the headteacher, who flew off the handle and accused us of being unwilling to accept the simple facts about Adam's diagnosis and what he could and couldn't do. It was shocking and humiliating, and even Gemma, always matter of fact and professional, had to fight hard to hold back the tears. The SENDCo privately phoned that evening to apologise and say she had never seen parents spoken to in such a way. Which was nice of her and made us feel less gaslighted, but seeing as she was apologising for her boss, presumably without his knowledge, it was rather a non-apology.

Many parents of *Zappas* will have sat through meetings like this and had similarly horrific experiences. They will have had to sit there while miserable news is delivered as though it's in their child's best interests. (Sometimes it is, but many times it isn't.) Like us, they'll have argued that reasonable adjustments should be made for the benefit of their child and been told they just don't get it. (Again, occasionally parents won't get it, but this needs to be dealt with in a compassionate way.) They'll have been made to feel powerless and humiliated. We certainly did.

In the end, after years of fighting, this was one battle we decided to leave. We were undoubtedly in the right and had the weight of law in our favour, but sometimes it feels like too much effort. We were almost done with primary school, and we had to weigh up whether our initial desire to take them on one last time was really born of the best of intentions or just to get one over on them. As it happens, when we sat down with Adam that evening and explained that he wasn't going on the trip, he wasn't particularly fussed. He would have had a good time but, like many children with autism, he does appreciate routine and would have missed his creature comforts. It was painful and we didn't want to accept it lying down, but this time we did. And each day of the residential we took Adam out for a trip of his own, including a fast-food lunch, so he felt like he'd had a special week regardless.

In this case, as in others, we were lucky to have Gemma's experience as a former SENDCo. However, I can imagine for most people these meetings are not just a time-suck but utterly bewildering and potentially traumatic. So here are a few tips to hopefully make the surfeit of meetings a little more manageable.

1. Be judicious about what requires a meeting and what doesn't

Having three *Zappas*, we've had to become more careful with our time and we've learnt to sometimes nope out. Some schools like meetings more than others, and often it's more about their accountability than what's right for you or your child. If you feel it isn't relevant or necessary, be prepared to follow the advice of Nancy Reagan and 'Just Say No'.

2. Be honest if you're too tired or overwhelmed

Don't forget, the likelihood is the teachers are parents too and they will hopefully understand. Due to the burden of all the meetings for Adam and Dylan, we've barely been to one at Zoe's school for the past five years. It could be they think we're the world's shittiest parents, and if that's the case so be it. We have our limits, and in truth I believe they're a good school and trust them to use their initiative and make the right decisions. Remember, just because a meeting is routine for them doesn't mean it's routine for you.

3. Do what you can to reduce the time involved

If you're working, be clear you can't simply drop everything at a moment's notice. Ask if the school would be prepared to move the meeting online or have a phone call instead. And if you must attend in person, there are several things you can do: try to schedule it after drop-off or before pick-up; ask for an agenda so that each minute is used properly; see if you can combine several meetings into one; and agree a time limit in advance. You may worry that your child's school will judge you, but ultimately a parent who values their time is a good parent.

4. Don't allow it to become confrontational

Even if you have a good relationship with your child's school, meetings can sometimes get fraught. Don't be afraid to stop a meeting if it's getting too much and you need some time to think. You don't need to feel pressured, so ask if you can have a break or arrange to reconvene another time. And don't act out of spite or because you want to believe you've won. Sometimes a battle isn't worth fighting and it's better to leave your powder dry for another day. Your child's well-being is all that really matters, not point-scoring. Three–nil to me for stressing that fact.

5. Don't go alone

These meetings can be difficult, so feel free to bring along a friend or relative for moral support. It doesn't matter whether they have a relationship with the school or not, this is your prerogative. You might also want to think about getting professional help. There's so much legislation and procedure to get your head around, which can be impenetrable for parents. Gemma's experience in schools has been invaluable for us, so consider finding a parent advocate. Alternatively, why not ask Gemma? She'll do it in exchange for a decaf latte from Starbucks and can be contacted via the publisher.

6. Bring your own biscuits

A clever loophole, this one. So long as you always turn up with a tin of McVitie's Family Circle, even if you walk in and find a box of tissues on the table, you've immediately turned it into a biscuits meeting instead. Plus being yours, you can make sure you bagsy the good ones. Nothing will ever seem too bad if you can make the SENDCo eat the digestives while you help yourself to the happy jam faces.

2

Q IS FOR QUESTIONABLE SOCIAL SKILLS

I am not entirely sure whether it's due to their needs or merely that they're Blakers, but my little and not so little *Zappas* don't really do social skills. I hesitate to say they have none at all, but if it's somehow possible to misjudge a situation, then our children can and will.

For a start, one trait my autistic boys have in common is they often take things entirely literally and can't read the nuance of a joke. Some years ago Dylan asked me whether the bright light in the sky was the moon or a plane. Knowing he'd believe anything, I replied, 'Neither, it's the Bat Signal.' I got my comeuppance immediately because his response was, 'Seriously?! Batman's in Edgware?! That's it, I'm not going to bed until I've seen him and got his autograph.'

I'd love to say that Dylan has got better in this area, but I'd be lying. Even as he approaches 15 years of age, he doesn't really get comedy. Which would be fine, except his father is a comedian. Yes, truthfully! So I'm forever biting my lip and trying to stop myself from making jokes in his presence. Sarcasm is especially problematic for an autistic child like Dylan. He was recently out on a Friday afternoon and texted me to ask what time I'd like him back. Being a world-renowned stand-up/annoying sarky dad, I replied, '6 p.m. on Monday'. Dylan responded, 'But it's Friday. Why are you saying Monday?' Hmmm, if you really want to know, it's precisely because of interactions like this one.

This isn't to say Dylan doesn't turn his own hand to comedy from time to time. Well, I say comedy, but I use that term rather loosely. This is surreal humour as filtered through Dylan's rather mystifying brain. One of his favourite current activities – when taking a short break from watching YouTube videos about how the government uses tattoos to track our movements – is to make memes from old photos of his father. Hey, everyone needs a hobby.

The most recent one featured yours truly from when I was a contestant on *University Challenge* in 1996. This was back when I had long hair and a beard and looked like a Jewish Jesus. Or Jesus, as that should be. There I am, sitting next to one of my teammates from Keble College, Oxford, but instead of our surnames – Blaker and Richards – Dylan has replaced them in the most rudimentary fashion with the words 'Penis' and 'Pussy'. This fits in with the title of the meme that's to be found in large block capitals above our heads. 'WHO WILL WIN? THE PENIS OR THE PUSSY?' I did say it was surreal.

I was genuinely baffled by this and asked Dylan if he was able to explain the joke. I present his explanation exactly as I received it.

It being *University Challenge*, you would expect the names to be proper, although the names of penis and pussy/vagina are humorous as they are words of funny genitalia. The punchline is then the title asking a rhetorical question of who will win, the penis or the pussy. This confirms the names of penis and pussy being accurate, and as they are not proper names, instead names of genitalia, this is funny.

There you have it. Personally, I think this is unfathomable nonsense, but then *Mrs. Brown's Boys* has run for over 11 years and won a BAFTA, so what do I know?

Of course, the tendency in the Blaker house to take everything literally means no one can get on because the boys accept every insult at face value. Some time ago Dylan was hysterical because Edward had said he was a panda who can't hop. He ran into my office demanding that I punish his brother.

'Hang on, are you a panda?' I asked.

'No.'

'Good. And can you hop?'

Dylan demonstrated his hopping prowess. Nothing amazing, but clearly he could hop, and he answered 'yes'.

'OK, not a problem then. Shut the door on your way out.'

Barely a week later Dylan was the perpetrator, this time doing the name-calling and causing Edward to disturb me with a similar grievance. He burst into my bedroom crying because Dylan had called him an abacus.

'Are you an abacus?' I asked him wearily.

He looked at me blankly.

'OK, let me ask you a different question. What is an abacus?'

Again, he looked confused. 'I don't know.'

'Well, if you don't know what it is, how do you know you don't want to be one? Maybe being an abacus is the greatest thing in the world. Maybe it's cool.'

This made Edward looked particularly dubious. 'No one says "cool" anymore. It's "sick".' And at that he wandered off, laughing at his father's utter unhipness.

Unfortunately, all this 'You're a panda who can't hop' and 'You're an abacus' is just the charming younger phase of my children's social ineptitude. After they hit puberty it starts to go downhill fast. Adam took eight years to learn to speak, but on becoming a teenager took eight minutes to learn to swear. Were conversations with him bleeped, it would sound like we were living with R2-D2, which would probably be Edward's idea of heaven.

At 16, Adam genuinely insisted that we refer to him by his rap name, which is MC Sex Offender. Frighteningly, he thought being known as MC Sex Offender made him sound really cool rather than an R Kelly tribute act. The only name that could be worse is if he called himself MC Prince Andrew. Now he's 14, Dylan too has started to think it's cool – I mean sick – to speak mostly in hip hop-styled patois. He recently did his end of Year 9 exams and I asked him how his English paper went. He simply looked at me and did that arms-crossed gesture – you know, the one that if you're a teenage white boy makes you look like an utter twat – then replied, 'Bitchin'!' I guess I'll have to wait for his results to find out whether that means they went well or badly.

But that's the thing with having few social skills: you don't have a filter and will say whatever comes into your head no matter how inappropriate. And if Buckingham Palace didn't like that joke about Prince Andrew, then that's my excuse too. A few years ago Adam went on a school trip – yes, his secondary school let him go without any arguments! – and we were very excited for his return, so we could hear how he got on. The little ones made 'Welcome Home' signs for the front door, and we were all ready to make a big fuss of him. However, when he entered the house, before we even got the chance to ask about his week in North Wales, he had one question on his mind.

'Dad, have you heard of golden showers?'

I looked at him, probably slightly puzzled (not standing in front of a mirror, I couldn't see my own face. I could ask Adam for his recollection, but having autism – and so being largely unable to read social cues – I'd be surprised if he'd be able to confirm one way or the other).

'Yes, Adam. Why do you ask?'

He replied matter-of-factly, 'Nothing. What's for supper?'

And that was that, we moved on. I never did find out why this had popped into his head and, more pertinently, what exactly he'd seen on this school trip that had prompted his urolagnia-themed enquiry.

Communication has never been Adam's strong suit. I still have a scar on my forehead from the time he appeared at the door of my office, threw an Argos catalogue at me and snarled, 'You know I like football, so where are my goalposts?' After briefly checking myself for signs of concussion, I managed to deduce that Adam had found some pictures of goalposts, and this was his way of saying he'd be grateful if I invested my hard-earned money on buying them for the garden. All that, plus a side order of reproach for me failing to read his mind and purchasing them already.

Obviously, I was rather annoyed with Adam. I do accept that one day I'll die, but this wasn't the way I wanted to go. I can't tell you how happy I was when, in 2020, Argos discontinued what Bill Bailey called the 'Book of Dreams'. For me it was more a 'Book of Nightmares', and in going online only it at least ended the possibility of me falling victim to homicide by Argos catalogue.* Yet it says a lot that at the time of the incident now known in our house as 'Argosgate' I was so happy that Adam would communicate at all, I was prepared to totally overlook the fact that it came alongside GBH with an 800-page book. This is what parenting a child with autism can do to you. In more ways than one, it really does move the goalposts. And if that's not a dad joke, I don't know what is!

Meanwhile, Zoe's social skills aren't much better, and in her case I can't even put it down to inherited Blaker belligerence. Perhaps during her 12 years of living with us she has acquired it by osmosis. Zoe can be incredibly stubborn and contrary. Not in the way my other teens are, of course. I recently took away Dylan's pocket money as punishment for calling Edward a dick, and he insisted that while he accepted it was wrong, the amount of money he was losing was far greater than the crime

---

* Granted, Adam could bring up the website on his laptop and then hurl that at me, but it wouldn't be the same. This would be Death by Chromebook, which is totally different.

merited. With a limited vocabulary and understanding, Zoe is more basic in her argumentativeness. She reminds me of the sketch in *Monty Python's Flying Circus* where Michael Palin pays John Cleese to have an argument with him.

'Look, this isn't an argument.'

'Yes, it is.'

'No, it isn't, it's just contradiction.'

'No, it isn't.'

'Yes, it is.'

Tell Zoe it's bedtime and she'll reply, 'No, not bedtime!' Ask her to come for a bath and she'll respond, 'iPad, not bath.' Ask her to come to the table for dinner and she'll counter, 'Not dinner, breakfast.' Frustratingly, she'll even contradict herself. I can tell her we're going to the park, and she'll answer, 'Not park, home'; and then an hour later, when I tell her it's time to leave the park will say, 'Not home, park.' I have been tempted to sit Zoe down and use Michael Palin's line: 'An argument is an intellectual process. Contradiction is just the automatic gainsaying of anything the other person says.' Sadly, I don't think she'd get the reference.

She's so stroppy she'll even argue about things that have nothing to do with her. If I ever tell The Bailey to be quiet – I'll be honest, it's a regular occurrence – Zoe will pipe up with, 'No, let Bailey speak.' She's like the voice of God, sitting quietly watching her iPad or drawing, and every so often chipping in with lines like, 'No, let Edward have ketchup' or 'No, give Dylan his pocket money.'

'But Zoe,' I'll say, 'he called Edward a dick. That's very naughty!'

'No, dick not naughty.' And on it goes.

Sometimes the bolshiness isn't even about something in the present. Zoe has the most remarkable memory and will frequently be obstinate in relation to a seemingly trivial incident that happened months or even years earlier. About six years ago, while Zoe was in the bath, we had a power cut and all the lights went out. She was understandably scared being in the pitch black, and while no child would like that, it took nearly half a decade for Zoe to stop mentioning it every single day. 'No bath, don't want dark!' She still goes on about the day the school bus had a broken windscreen wiper – 'Don't want bus, wipers not working' – and we must coax her on board by showing her that they're perfectly operational.

The only times she uses more complex phrases are when she repeats sentences she's heard at school. The result is we get a fascinating insight into what goes on in the classroom. Some of these lines are self-explanatory: 'What a day!' or 'Good boy, Danny'. On other occasions, they're more esoteric and require further investigation. For example, there was a time Zoe, completely out the blue, declared, 'Only vegetables, not arms!' She said this several more times before we put the pieces together. Have you worked it out for yourself? If you've not deduced it yet, it seems there must have been a biting incident in class, and the culprit was told that if there's any munching going on, it needs to be 'only vegetables, not arms'. My money is on Danny because since becoming a Blaker, Zoe's diet is now almost entirely free of vegetables. Had the line been 'Only crisps, not arms' I'd have been a bit more concerned.

Except for these parroted phrases, Zoe isn't the most natural conversationalist. Ask her what she's doing and

I'd wager the money in my pocket that her response will be, 'Nuffing.'* It doesn't matter what the enquiry is:

'Zoe, what did you do in school today?'

'Zoe, do you need to go to the toilet?'

'Zoe, what are you watching?' (I can see with my own eyes what she's watching, and she can see that I can see what she's watching, but she'll still almost certainly reply, 'Nuffing.')

Even if the question is, 'Zoe, what do you want for lunch?' it's 50/50 whether the answer will be 'chips' or 'nuffing'. It is such a likelihood that any interaction with Zoe will prompt her to say 'nuffing', that it's become one of Adam's favourite pastimes. He spends much of the day asking Zoe completely random questions to see if he can get her to reply 'nuffing' for his own amusement. All teenagers need to let their hair down, and trying to make a child with Down syndrome say her catchphrase is both preferable to drugs and substantially cheaper. And while it's arguably cruel to use a child with SEN for sport, I put this down as one of those things that I couldn't do myself, but for which Adam has special licence.

Sadly, Adam's baiting of his sister is merely the tip of the iceberg when it comes to interactions between my children, as their dubious social skills make our house like a tinderbox. Some would suggest this is due to the frankly ludicrous number of kids we have, but my great-grandparents had many children too and their homes didn't look like mine. It's saying something that I now look enviously at my ancestors crammed into unsanitary

---

* Don't get too excited. I don't have any money in my pocket, and these days I pretty much only use Apple Pay. Sorry!

accommodation in 19th-century Russia. They may have dealt with poverty, disease and huge infant mortality, but I reckon I'm dealing with a much greater trauma. For a start, my forebears didn't have to adjudicate constant fights over screens and, even worse, chargers. There are times I lie in bed at the end of a long day and all I hear in my ears, like a terrible case of tinnitus, are repeated echoes of 'Dad, I need a new charger! Dad, I need a new charger! Dad, I need a new charger!'

Six children in the 21st century means a lot of phones, iPads, Nintendos and other devices, all of which require a charger that will inevitably get lost or broken within a week. We now have more useless technology in our house than the Virgin Media warehouse. I think chargers have become a bigger commodity in the Blaker family than money. The street value of a lightning cable in our house is currently double the cost in an Apple Store, and Adam is making a fortune loaning them out to the younger children at exorbitant prices. Underage wage slaves in China can't make these cables fast enough to satiate our need for chargers. Life expectancy in the European shtetl may have been only 35 years, but the life expectancy of a phone cable in our house isn't even 35 days, with a terrifying mortality rate of 25 per cent in the first week of their life. Perhaps this is just a curse of the modern age, and I shouldn't be surprised. However, I'd like to think that if only the children were able to communicate with each other in a more civilised way, then at least half those cables wouldn't have been snapped in USB-themed tugs of war.

Having read the first chapter, you may at this point be expecting some handy tips for what to do if you also have *Zappas* with questionable social skills. Sorry to disappoint, but while many of the upcoming chapters do conclude with advice, it's not going to be possible every time. This is just how our children are made, and I'm not sure what counsel I can offer beyond:

- Don't make sarcastic jokes they won't understand.
- Hide old photos of yourself so they can't turn them into memes.
- Always wear a helmet in case a catalogue gets thrown at your head.

Yet even without any bullet points of guidance, I hope this snapshot of my family life makes you realise you aren't alone. There are many of us living with children like this. Perhaps, having previously believed your children were a bit unsocialised, you're now feeling smug that at least they have more social skills than mine! And if that's the case, you're very welcome.

3

D IS FOR DIAGNOSIS
AUTISM

Our journey with our eldest son Adam was one that many readers will recognise. After experiencing a miscarriage 14 months earlier we were so excited to have our first child, and those early years should have been joyous. To be blunt, they turned into a nightmare.

There's a famous essay about the experience of having a child with SEN called 'Welcome to Holland'. The central premise is you were expecting to fly out for a holiday in Italy, and for some reason the plane lands instead in Holland. Or put another way, you were planning to listen to Coldplay's *A Rush of Blood to the Head* but found yourself listening to Frank Zappa's *Hot Rats*. I bet the author, Emily Perl Kingsley, is kicking herself that she didn't think of that metaphor.* Anyway, this was very much us: anticipating one thing and being given another. Although to be honest, I think Holland sounds too nice for the analogy to truly work. And actually, I'd rather go

---

* In fairness, when she wrote 'Welcome to Holland' in 1987, Chris Martin was only ten.

to the Netherlands than Italy if given a choice.* I would say a more accurate description of our experience was that we had expected to go to Marbella and ended up in Kabul.

From the moment Adam came back from the hospital, he screamed continually and nothing would settle him. As naive new parents we assumed this was the norm. We put it down to everything from hunger and colic to teething and distress that Liverpool hadn't won the league for 14 years (the poor boy had to wait until he was nearly 16 for that last one to be put right). But none of these appeared to be the problem, at least not the first three, and no matter what formula we put him on and what reflux medicine he was prescribed, nothing seemed to alleviate his distress. He baffled doctors and midwives, and all we could do was hold on to the hope that surely at some point this would end. It had to. No one could be expected to live like this.

Yet if anything, it got worse. When Adam was 18 months old he was invited to his very first birthday party. Our neighbour's daughter was turning two, and they were hosting a tea with games in the garden. What a delightful way to spend an afternoon, we thought. We were really looking forward to it but became somewhat disheartened as the party unfolded. Adam didn't want to run around shrieking with the other children – strange, because as a rule running around shrieking was one of his favourite activities – preferring to sit in a deserted living room, pushing a car back and forth on the same

---

* Note to my editor: if this book gets translated into Italian, please remove this line.

stretch of carpet. I think deep down Gemma and I already knew there were some issues with Adam, but this was the first time the penny really dropped, so we started seeking professional help.

It would be a year and a half until a paediatrician formally diagnosed him as autistic, informing us that he scored appropriately on nearly all the categories of diagnostic rating, including obsessions, rigidity, speech delay and sensory issues. However, by this point it was hardly a surprise as we had ourselves joined the dots together. The main concern was that Adam wasn't talking. We knew his severely delayed and disordered development of language skills alone fulfilled the criteria for a formal diagnosis of childhood autism. On top of that, he ate almost nothing except bread, pasta and sweets. He required support to use a fork and mostly ate with his fingers if he was feeling polite, alternatively just putting his face in the bowl. He showed no signs of wanting to use the toilet or even indicating when he was dirty. He hated any change from his normal routine, crying hysterically when we tried cleaning him in the bathroom rather than on his changing table. He only wore short sleeves, would cover his ears to avoid loud sounds and insisted on having two of everything so he could carry one item in each hand. When he wasn't holding his toys in his left and right palm, he was lining them up, especially the many *Thomas and Friends* trains we bought him as rewards for almost any minor achievement. He hid his face and refused to give eye contact to anyone who spoke to him. He'd had a few playdates with other children, but none ever led to an attachment. Basically, he would only do anything on his own terms; or put another way, he was a Blaker.

It's hard to express how tough these years were for me and Gemma. After that fateful birthday party, Adam was referred to a local speech and language therapy service, where he saw a speech therapist for one-on-one sessions. He also joined a weekly early language group followed by an attention and listening group. And so we had an instant introduction to two recurring themes in our lives as parents of *Zappas*: endless meetings and hospital appointments.

We also had such a variety of experts visiting our home, we really needed a revolving door. Every time I looked up there was someone else observing Adam while furiously scribbling notes on a clipboard. There was the SALT (speech and language therapist) from the local council's tracker project; the council's pre-school teacher; a family support worker; the area SENDCo; teachers from BEAM (Barnet Early Autism Model); and specialists in something called TEACCH. It apparently stands for Teaching, Expanding, Appreciating, Collaborating and Cooperating with colleagues, and Holistic, and if I'd needed to tell you that without the help of Google I'd still be guessing next year. When it comes to abbreviations, it's up there with SPLINK, the mnemonic slogan from a 1970s public information film about road safety starring Jon Pertwee, which was so unmemorable that by the time you'd recalled what it stood for you'd almost certainly been run over.

All these professionals would watch Adam playing while shaking their heads and making tutting sounds, like builders considering a bad job you wanted them to fix. 'Tut tut tut, you've had cowboys in here. No speech, disordered social skills, sensory issues. Tut tut tut. This is going to cost you!!'

Even more problematic was Adam's behaviour. He was clearly unhappy and would spend an incredible amount of time crying. His lack of speech made it hard for him to communicate and so he resorted to a variety of attention-seeking habits, including kicking, biting and hitting. He'd run around the house, jump on furniture and loved turning himself upside down. Especially challenging for us was Adam's lack of any awareness of safety. He required constant supervision as he only needed a couple of seconds to put himself at risk. We'd think he was playing in the garden, but then he'd escape down the side entrance and we'd only realise when he'd ring on the doorbell to come back inside. We get so many people knocking to ask if we'd like our windows cleaned or paving re-laid, it's a miracle we didn't ignore him. On other occasions he'd spot the front door open – probably to tell someone we don't want our drive jet-sprayed, thank you very much – and he'd high tail it past us and run up the street, or even worse into the road. The word 'Stop' had no effect and neither did he have any interest when I tried to teach him the Green Cross Code. Probably because for the life of me, I could never remember what SPLINK stood for.

The scariest incident was the time I took our then two boys to the high street and Adam, who always refused to hold our hands, legged it into a butcher's shop. Not content with just browsing the selection of sausages and frozen chickens, he ran behind the counter where meat was being sliced on a machine, while I tried to extract him before he could be turned into carpaccio. I finally managed to drag him out, kicking and screaming, while Ollie remained unattended in his buggy on the street. Thankfully we got away with it, and I immediately bought a double buggy so that in the future Adam would be safely strapped in and couldn't try to start an apprenticeship in our local Dewhurst.

Had someone made off with Ollie while he was left unguarded, he would at least have been spared the years as Adam's punchbag. Being so close in age, they always had a very close relationship, and Ollie looked up to his older brother and wanted to spend as much time with him as possible. This meant the job of protecting him was all the more difficult since any time we tried to separate the boys, Ollie would be bereft at being parted from his abuser. He thought he was flying to Rome but ended up going to Stockholm.

Our best tactic for stopping the rough play was to constantly find stuff to do with them, whether it was trips to the park or carrying out chores. But that either involved interaction with other children – see 'F is for Friendships' and 'I is for Ignoring the Idiots' to understand why we might have wanted to avoid that – or heading to the shops and risking a repeat of 'Butchergate'. I usually opted for supermarkets, the aisles of which would at least accommodate our whopping double buggy, and which the boys always enjoyed, even though Adam had usually opened every food packet by the time we reached the checkout.

With Adam's behaviour unpredictable at best, we also retreated further into our own world. It didn't seem fair to put him in situations that would be challenging for him, so we spent years refusing invitations to almost all social gatherings. We'd only recently moved to a new area and had hoped to make local friends. Sadly, this didn't happen as we naturally put Adam first, even if it was to our detriment. Please let it go on record that this was the sole reason Gemma and I didn't make any friends in our community, and it was absolutely nothing to do with me being a curmudgeonly bastard.

If the days were tough, the evenings were even harder. Adam didn't seem to understand that nights are for sleeping and would often wake around midnight ready to play. He'd run around the house turning on lights and waking everyone up. Unsurprisingly, after spending the wee small hours demanding I play with him, he was regularly sent home from nursery for being unable to keep his eyes open. He was essentially operating in his own time zone: AMT, Adam Mean Time.

Upsettingly, Adam also appeared to have a complete lack of empathy and struggled to read social situations, both at nursery and at home. He would watch someone cry and not understand why. When Ollie sobbed, Adam would more often than not just laugh, especially worrying since more often than not he was the cause of the tears. Gemma was particularly upset when one day she fell down the stairs in front of the boys. She was lying on the floor in agony, thinking she may have broken her hip. As one might expect, Ollie was very distressed seeing his mother in such pain. Meanwhile, Adam just pointed and giggled away to himself. It was as though he were a proto-Jeremy Beadle, sniggering in the background while his victim falls prey to his plan. 'What Mummy doesn't know is that I've left some toys on the landing which she's going to trip on. Let's see if she's "Game for a Laugh"!'

Of course he didn't say anything of the sort. If only he had, because I'm sure much of Adam's behaviour had its root in his communication issues. Reports at the time suggested he displayed communicative intent and had reasonably good comprehension, but with hardly any expressive language he became extremely frustrated. His only words at this point were 'Dadda', which was me, and 'Babba', which was Ollie. What a cuss on Gemma: not only did he laugh when she fell down the stairs, he didn't even have the good grace to say 'Mama'.

With the encouragement of some of the many professionals in our house, we started teaching Adam PECS. This is short for Picture Exchange Communication System and is essentially a series of cards designed to allow autistic children to convey their thoughts and needs. Typically, Adam waited for us to make cards for his favourite foods – given he only ate bread, pasta and sweets, at least it wasn't too much effort – and for all the toys in our playroom, before developing his own hand gestures, thus prompting the experts to suggest we abandon PECS in favour of Makaton.* I think he was just determined to make our lives as challenging as possible. So predictably, no sooner had we invested in a guidebook to Makaton that Adam started speaking. I think it was only the fact we already owned all the Makaton resources

---

* If you aren't aware of it, Makaton is a language programme that uses symbols, signs and speech to enable people to communicate. You might have seen Justin Fletcher use it as Mr Tumble on the BBC series *Something Special* and assumed he was doing tic-tac like John McCririck on *Channel 4 Racing*. Nope, this is Makaton.

and wanted to put them to good use that encouraged us to adopt a child with Down syndrome four years later.

During this awfully trying period, there were many times Gemma and I wondered if we'd made a massive mistake having Ollie so soon after Adam. Did having a new-born to look after mean Adam wasn't getting the attention he needed? Was Ollie also getting a raw deal by being subjected to Adam's love for rough and tumble? Yet for all the doubts, I remain convinced this was real serendipity. I know serendipity means happy accident, so if you're reading this, Ollie, I didn't intend it like that. I meant more that having a younger brother, one who was technically a *Coldplay*, was a real benefit to Adam. For example, there was always someone else with whom we could practise sharing, and we even bought a sand timer so Adam would know when it was his turn. Would that have been possible without having a willing sibling to join in?

Likewise, while I'm sure the numerous SALT sessions helped, and I don't want to minimise anyone's work with Adam, his language truly developed when he learnt new words from his younger brother. I should stress that he was still only intelligible to those who spoke 'Adam Blaker', and even C-3PO, fluent in over six million forms of communication, would most likely have been stumped. Among his admittedly small vocabulary were:

Bo – ball
Boo – blue
D – dog
Ka – cat
Do – go (but sometimes Play-Doh)

Pa-ah – pasta
Cho – chocolate
Cri – crips
Ebra – zebra
Elba – elbow (but possibly also a request to watch
    Luther)

OK, so he wasn't quite Stephen Fry, but Rome wasn't built in a day, and it brought me and Gemma great joy to hear Adam finally speaking and telling us what he wanted. The future suddenly seemed a hell of a lot rosier.

But do you want to know the thing that cheered us the most during this period? It was when the paediatrician finally diagnosed Adam as autistic. Perhaps that sounds crazy to some readers. For many, hearing the news of a diagnosis, whether for autism or anything else, would be a devastating blow, confirming all their worst fears for their child. For us, however, this was a moment of serenity: at last, professional confirmation that we weren't just imagining Adam's issues, nor were we merely shit parents who couldn't cope and were failing our son.

I can't overstate how important this realisation was to me and Gemma. It may appear obvious when written down, but it's hard sometimes to remember that parenting is not a chance to show the world you're a success. For the first three years of his life I think we both felt that if Adam failed, then we'd failed; that in falling behind his peers, we must have done something wrong. Maybe I'd spent too long watching football when I should have been playing educational games with my son and showing him flashcards. I'd almost certainly spent too long watching football, but that wasn't the cause of Adam's issues, and now I had a piece of paper to prove it.

In truth we shouldn't have needed a diagnosis to bring this realisation. We should have already understood that as much as we loved our child, he wasn't the measure of our self-worth. He didn't reflect anything about us: he is who he is, and we are who we are. So, whether you have a letter from a doctor or not, let me save you years of self-recrimination and misery right now. If you have a child like Adam – or any child, come to think of it – stop taking sole responsibility for their destiny because that's exhausting and untenable. In fact, you're stealing something that doesn't belong to you. You're taking over their journey, and no one likes a back-seat driver.

Somehow, the definition of success in parenting has become whether your children turn out exactly like you. But to release yourself from this way of thinking is to release yourself from a lifetime of frustration and disappointment if your children fail to comply with your plans. My children failed to comply from day one. But so long as you provide unconditional love, a safe environment away from meat-slicing machines, and unlimited pa-ah, cho and cri, you've fulfilled everything you need to do, and you can wave them off, short sleeves and all.

Six years later we went through this all again when Dylan received a diagnosis. By this point we didn't need a letter from a psychiatrist to comprehend our lives but, interestingly, I feel Dylan did. OK, perhaps not at six years old, but as he approached his teens I know it explained the many ways in which he felt different. People who receive a diagnosis of autism in adulthood often say they wish they'd known earlier, as it would have helped them navigate their way through traumatic parts of their childhood. When I asked my third son about this, he told me he's aware that he has many hyperfixations, from *The Simpsons* to *Batman*, hates maintaining eye contact for more than 20 seconds and struggles in many of his lessons at school. And this all makes sense to him because he knows he's autistic. We all have a need to understand who we are and those with autism are no different. In Dylan's words, 'It's why I feel a bit weird.'

If someone literally expected to be going to Italy and then ended up in Holland, it will probably have been their own cock-up. They'd have either got on the wrong plane – not sure how that could happen as they check your boarding pass, but let's go with it – or they just weren't paying attention when they booked the ticket. It wouldn't have been your fault if you got on a plane to Rome and terrorists demanded it be rerouted to Amsterdam, but I don't think that's what's happening in this metaphor. If you were the victim of a hijack, you'd be much more concerned about being held captive on a plane rather than the fact you wound up holidaying in the Netherlands. Plus, the hijackers I've seen on screen tend to prefer places like Cuba. I've never watched a movie where armed guerrillas hold the cabin crew hostage until they get to visit the Anne Frank Museum.

That's why this analogy is so annoying. Having a child with SEN is not your fault. It's not your mistake. It's not a judgement on your parenting. It's just one of those things. I'm not sure what would be a better simile. I was expecting to rent a video starring Bruce Lee, but I've come back from Blockbusters with a movie starring Bruce Li. I wanted to book Mark Chapman from *Match of the Day*, but booked the bloke who killed John Lennon. I was planning to go to Italy, then someone in China ate something in a market and I've spent the best part of a year home schooling my kids. None of them quite work. This was more: I was expecting to raise Adam Blaker and ended up raising Adam Blaker. That's basically the nub of it.

If you find yourself struggling with a young child who isn't progressing as you think they should, here are a few tips to keep in mind.

1. Seek intervention early

Don't worry about the stigma of working with speech and language therapists or your child being labelled. Just listen to your gut instinct. If you feel something is wrong, get professional help. Whether it leads to a diagnosis or not, there are so many resources to tap into, so don't wait.

2. It will get better!!

These early years were awful, but Adam did grow up. He learnt to speak (admittedly mostly swear words); he made friends (admittedly other *Zappas* who wanted to destroy our home); he improved his diet (admittedly only broadened to McDonald's, Nando's and KFC); and he stopped laughing when I hurt myself. Well, sometimes.

3. Motivation, motivation, motivation

If you have a child like Adam, they will probably want to do everything on their own terms. But this doesn't mean you won't be able to find motivation that works for them. We tried it all, from star charts to tactical ignoring to rewarding with treats. Some worked better than others, but it's got to be worth a go.

4. Ignore other people

More on this to come later in the book, but I wish we'd realised this sooner. Taking Adam everywhere in a double buggy seemed to cause others to disapprove and even avoid us. Why would a child his age still need a buggy?! Just do what you have to and what works for your child. Everyone else can sod off.

5. Not everyone needs a label

It may be that you decide not to pursue a diagnosis. We have children whom we felt wouldn't particularly benefit from heading down this path. If they wish to seek one in their adult life they can, but for now they exist perfectly happily without a label.

6. If you do receive a diagnosis, embrace it

It's not bad news. It's merely confirmation of what you may have already suspected and means you can now unlock much more help. It could also be good news for your child; many late-diagnosed autistic adults say they wish they'd known as kids, as it would have saved them years of trauma trying to understand why they were different.

7. Remember, this isn't your fault

This is nothing to do with whether you played them Tchaikovsky or showed them flashcards. Life has merely thrown you a curveball. You were expecting to go to Italy and guess what: you've ended up in Italy. Maybe the weather is a bit shit and the queue at passport control is far too long due to Brexit, but you're where you wanted to be all the time. Just hold on a few days, the weather's going to get better.

4

X IS FOR X-RAYS AND OTHER HOSPITAL APPOINTMENTS

The excessive school meetings are annoying, but as time sucks go they have nothing on the countless hospital visits. On top of the autism and Down syndrome, between our children there is ADHD, speech and language disorders, heart conditions, hearing loss, mobility issues, sensory needs and gastroenterological problems. You know you've got a lot going on when Great Ormond Street give you your own parking space.

Zoe accounts for most of these appointments on her own. When we started down the long road towards adopting her in 2010, we really had no idea quite how much would be involved. Like many children with Down syndrome she was born with an atrioventricular septal defect (AVSD), a large hole in the centre of her heart that required open heart surgery almost immediately. Of course, at this point in her short life we were completely unaware of her existence so didn't go through the incredible trauma this would have brought. But while we didn't suffer that anguish, the operation wasn't the end of it and Zoe has needed annual check-ups with heart specialists ever since.

Possibly worrying that we'd missed out on the surgery in Zoe's infancy, in 2013 the consultant informed us that the hole in her heart had widened and so there would have to be a sequel: *Heart Op II: The Endocardial Cushion Strikes Back*. I can joke now because thankfully Zoe came through it and recovered incredibly quickly, but it was no laughing matter at the time. Before we even arrived at the hospital, the doctor matter-of-factly informed us there was a real possibility of death. And even that was nothing to the cold reality of seeing our daughter, post-surgery, lying in bed with so many different coloured tubes exiting her body that we had half a mind to call the bomb squad. The only positive was they made it very hard to see her torso, so we didn't immediately notice the enormous scar that ran from her collar bone to her stomach.*

Zoe still has a frankly unreasonable number of appointments, but they have at least decreased since she first moved into our home. At that point she had weekly occupational therapy to help with her low muscle tone; regular visits to the cardiologist about her heart; back to the hospital for the ENT department to test her hearing; and then back again to see the ophthalmologist to monitor her eyes. We should've gone to Specsavers, but alas that wasn't offered since they don't deal with cataracts, strabismus or the world's least cooperative two-year-old. Even things mums and dads normally take for granted, such as taking their child to the shoe shop, which admittedly can be traumatic for parents of the most

---

* See the photo in 'E is for Embarrassing Photos'. Though this one isn't embarrassing, it's fucking scary.

well-behaved *Coldplay*, required an appointment at the orthotics department. I've sat in so many hospital waiting rooms that if I ever go on *Celebrity Mastermind* my specialist subject will be back issues of *Heat* magazine.

Probably the most challenging hospital visits in recent years have been Zoe's gastro appointments. For as long as we've known her, Zoe has had what can only be described as unspeakable constipation. She can go several days without doing anything and is more backed up than the M25. Having poor communication, she isn't able to express how this makes her feel, but it's usually pretty evident from her general demeanour. After a week of inactivity, poor Zoe will be crying and very unhappy, so naturally we've kept asking to see consultants to try to work out what is going on with her stomach. As a result, she's been prodded and X-rayed more times than I can remember, and we've had the joy of administering all manner of foods, powders and medications.

One of strangest jobs was overseeing a shape test, otherwise known as a Bowel Transit Study. Before I go any further, let me check that you're not eating anything at the moment. If you are, I suggest putting this book down until you've finished. If not, then I'll start and try to keep this as brief as possible. The shape test is basically an examination to find out how long it takes for poo to pass through the colon. In practice, this meant getting Zoe to eat three capsules, each filled with ten small white plastic shapes, on three successive days. The idea is that these shapes – circles, squares and rectangles – would pass through her bowel and then, seeing as she was bunged up, would be visible on an X-ray a week later. The key question for the doctors was how far down her tummy would they be by the time they looked. However, the key question for us was how on earth would we get Zoe to eat these flipping capsules.

Swallowing them like pills was completely out the question for her, so the next step was to follow the doctor's advice and empty the shapes into a yoghurt. There was only one small flaw: Zoe doesn't like yoghurt. She likes chips. Sometimes she'll eat spaghetti and sometimes she'll stick to bread, but mostly she wants chips. Which is fine – well, it isn't fine, but this isn't the chapter about food, that's coming later – but one issue is the shapes can't be emptied onto chips. Obviously they can, but even Zoe, with her poor sight and lazy eye, would spot them immediately and either brush them straight off or, more likely, scream the house down until we remade the chips from scratch.

The best option we could think of was ice cream, because even the ever-fussy Zoe won't turn this down. Her favourite is chocolate, but I worried those white shapes would be too obvious, so for our nefarious purposes it had to be vanilla. It also needed to be pains-takingly melted to be just the right consistency at the precise moment that we wanted her to eat it. Not too solid that the shapes wouldn't be easily mixed in; but not too runny that it became impossible for Zoe to eat it. I felt like an alchemist, trying to turn Ben & Jerry's base metal into Ben & Jerry's gold. Or as Ben & Jerry's would probably call it 'Bold Cold Gold', in this case topped off with deli-cious plastic shapes instead of the usual cookie bites.

I'd love to tell you this huge effort was worth it, but I can't say it was. The study did work in one sense, because when I took Zoe back to the hospital for her X-ray I could clearly see the shapes in her stomach. The inside of her belly looked like a handbag into which someone had emptied Smarties, Tic Tacs and Chewits. Some shapes were lower down, approaching the exit, and others were higher up, as though they were in the middle of her ribcage. Most were on the right, but then some were on the left. I took a photo of the X-ray on the monitor to show Gemma, but then got told off by the nurses who said this wasn't allowed. I'd have thought as a parent – and the poor sod who'd spent three days liquifying ice cream – that I'd have had every right to take a photo, but they were quite insistent I stop and delete the one I'd already taken.*

Examining the X-ray, I couldn't honestly make heads or tails of it and may as well have been looking inside a handbag of confectionery for all it told me. Which was fine because I'm a comedian not a gastroenterologist. But you know what the specialist said? What incredible wisdom he'd gleaned from what he'd seen on the screen? That the shapes proved that Zoe was badly constipated. No shit, Sherlock. Or rather, lots of shit, all of it with shapes in, stuck inside her tummy, Sherlock. So that was three days of melting ice cream and hiding the shapes; a trip to the hospital; and the usual struggles to get our uncooperative daughter to lie flat on the bed, all for them to tell us something I could have told you from the comfort of my sofa.

Remarkably, at this point things took a turn for the worse. Having successfully administered the shape study

---

* Not only did I merely pretend to delete the picture, but I now present it in 'E is for Embarrassing Photos'. Yeah, I'm a rebel!

ourselves, the consultant clearly felt he needed to up the ante to see what we could cope with. He now introduced us to a word I'd not heard of before but which still gives me nightmares. Disimpaction.

I know I only just asked if you were eating, but please allow me to check again because this really isn't pretty. Ready? OK, I did warn you. Disimpaction involves clearing out the bowel of all the retained stools. But rather than doing it in hospital, this was another do-it-yourself job. We were given strict instructions about how to follow a disimpaction regime, during which we'd feed Zoe laxatives in increasingly larger doses to 'clear out' all the accumulated poo. On Monday she'd have four sachets of Movicol in her orange juice, then on Tuesday it would be six, on Wednesday it would be eight, working up until the end of the week, when she'd have 12 sachets at once. Considering she'd previously had one sachet a day, I was briefly concerned that this could cause Zoe to OD on Movicol.

This, however, was the least of our worries because the specialist had a few other words of warning before sending us off. He said the goal was to completely empty her intestine of the backlog of poo, and we shouldn't stop increasing the laxatives until she was passing only brown water. Don't moan, I've warned you twice already. He stressed we needed to be prepared, advising us to stock up on toilet paper and wet wipes; to caution Zoe's siblings that the bathroom might be out of action; and, most alarmingly, to avoid letting Zoe anywhere near carpeted floors or fabric couches. Thanks a lot, doctor! And when can we come round and get shit stains all over your ottoman?

I was in two minds about including 'Disimpactiongate' in this book, not least in case you're squeamish, my dear reader. I've included it, though, because I think it's the perfect illustration of how parents of *Zappas* must often plug the resources gap in the underfunded NHS. Don't get me wrong, I'm aware that being a parent of a disabled child will frequently involve dealing with crap, both figuratively and literally. And trust me, I'm down for it. My gripe is that since specialists don't have the time to get their hands dirty – again, both figuratively and literally – they want us parents to do all the messy work instead. Ironically, I've heard physicians complain about patients who've made the mistake of consulting 'Dr Google' before going to a real doctor. But who can blame them when parents are asked to perform what is essentially medical DIY? Instructing me to take a week off work so I can feed Zoe a preposterous amount of laxative, and then be ready at any second to clear up the subsequent mess, is what us Jews would call *chutzpah*. Roughly translated it means 'a right fucking cheek', but somehow both less rude and ruder at the same time.

Us parents of children like Zoe have so many things to worry about. We live in fear concerning our children's health and have the burden of making potentially life or death decisions on a regular basis. And there's no question that the medical care in the NHS is, overall, outstanding. But considering the tremendous stress we all experience, what we need more than anything is someone to take over when it comes to shit like this (you guessed it, figuratively and literally). I know my strengths. I can fold clothes beautifully, reverse park a gigantic people carrier and have an encyclopaedic knowledge of

Hanna-Barbera cartoons.* I also know my limitations. I'm unable to touch my toes, can't speak any foreign languages and am crap at building flat-pack furniture. Likewise, I have no medical training, which is why this IKEA-style intervention felt equally daunting. 'Disimpactiongate' might as well have involved the doctor handing me an Allen key rather than 75 sachets of laxative.

Even when the medics are wonderful, the infrastructure and bureaucracy are enough to drive any parent to distraction. If you thought attending all the appointments was time-consuming, this is nothing compared with the job of *arranging* all the appointments. Having numerous children with special needs, I really need a PA whose sole job is to take this off my hands so I can perhaps, you know, do some work? Interestingly, none of the consultants, therapists or specialists ever get on the phone themselves. Why? Because they're doing their job. Unfortunately, most of us parents don't have this luxury and must get used to a life of constant interruption.

They call so that appointments can be made. Then they phone to say that they need to be rescheduled. At this point they'll explain that, for some unknown reason, a new date can't be offered on this call, and you'll have to wait for another call, which you can expect soon. (Spoiler alert: this is a very loose definition of the word 'soon'.) Eventually a new appointment will be made, and if you're lucky this one won't be rescheduled. However, they will

---

* If you meet me in the street, feel free to test me on *Scooby-Doo, Wacky Races, The Flintstones, Scooby's All-Star Laff-A-Lympics, Goober and the Ghost Chasers, Funky Phantom, Captain Caveman,* or *Help! ... It's the Hair Bear Bunch!*

call in advance to confirm that you can still make it, sometimes twice, perhaps thinking that on the first call you were lying.

One would like to imagine that through constantly dealing with families who have so much on their plate, hospital staff and other professionals would be extra-sensitive to the demands of our lives and make these interactions as pain-free as possible. Nice idea, anyway. I sometimes feel they go out of their way to employ only the most incompetent people available, just to test us that little bit more. Referral letters will be lost in the post. Prescriptions will have incomplete information, which will necessitate you having to ring to request replacements. And because they don't pick up the phone, you'll have to leave a message and wait months to be called back, which will inevitably happen at the most inconvenient time possible.

This is when you're lucky enough to have the correct number. Dylan has had to undergo several dental procedures at the Royal National ENT Hospital, who gave us both an incorrect phone number and email. It's a clever ploy if you don't want patients trying to reschedule their appointments. Most incredibly, when we were expecting our sixth (and final!) child the hospital gave us the wrong number to call for when Gemma entered labour. Her waters broke, and when I phoned the hospital to tell them we were on our way I got through to a local Domino's. The only delivery I was getting any help with was a Meat Feast with stuffed crust. I genuinely had to deliver the baby myself as she arrived before either the ambulance or my pizza had shown up. It was the most traumatic home delivery outside of Parcelforce. Knowing

The Bailey, she probably had something she needed to tell us, and it just couldn't wait, girlfriend.*

Even when we finally see the doctor, their computer never has any of the information they need. They spend the whole appointment explaining that their hospital uses a different system that doesn't sync with the local surgery, so sadly they don't have any of Zoe's records beyond 2007. Somehow my phone syncs with my iPad and laptop so I can always access every inane text message my mum has ever sent, yet no one is able to create a software package that enables healthcare professionals to obtain crucial information about our children.

Having said all this, in late 2019 the universe perhaps felt us parents weren't struggling enough already. And so along came COVID-19, and all these things that were previously a total ball ache were upgraded to being a complete and utter pain in the arse.† Everyone who lived through this period will have their own personal lowlights, and we'll deal with home schooling our SEN children later. But one thing everyone will remember is how quickly the pandemic became the catch-all excuse for poor customer service. It was suddenly impossible to contact your gas, mobile or internet provider, none of

---

* If you ever find yourself having to deliver a baby, let me reassure you it's not actually as hard as it sounds. It's a bit like facing a penalty in football. You could dive to your left or right, but there's a decent chance that it's going to come straight at you. So, stay where you are, make yourself as big as possible and you'll probably catch it easy enough.

† I realise some readers might prefer a pain in their testicles to one in their anus. Perhaps my years of suffering with haemorrhoids have made me fear bum ache more than anything else. Feel free to reverse these phrases if you wish.

which made enormous sense, because answering the phone in a call centre was precisely the kind of job that could easily move to the operators' own homes.

For me and Gemma, nowhere were these issues felt more keenly than regarding our children's appointments. It was understandable that hospital visits would be cancelled during a pandemic. What was harder to take was that it became impossible to reschedule any of these meetings; order repeat prescriptions; receive spare parts for a hearing aid; or any of the other myriad things that required speaking to a human being. Perhaps with the growing number of COVID cases it was all hands to the pump, but as stretched as hospitals were, surely patients with coronavirus weren't being treated by the reception-ist from children's orthotics. We joined the rest of the country in applauding NHS staff on Thursday evenings, but in my mind at least, I was excluding the admin staff who wouldn't reply to our emails or answerphone messages.

Things soon swung back the other way, and we were once more being bombarded with inconvenient daytime calls, all in the name of COVID protocols. Every appoint-ment was preceded by a phone conversation three days in advance to check whether anyone in the house had a temperature or been exposed to a positive case. And then again, one day in advance. And sometimes again on the day of the appointment, although perhaps it was just me they were targeting in revenge for being mentally excluded from my Thursday-night applause.

I don't want this chapter to be entirely negative, so, before we move on, here are some tricks I've discovered from my years attending hospital appointments. I can't make them all disappear from your diary, but I might be able to offer some quick wins that will help you feel a bit more positive. Because as any parent of a *Zappa* will appreciate, sometimes a quick win is the best we can hope for.

1. Leave plenty of time to get there

One thing I've learnt is you can't rush children with SEN. Whether you're going by car or public transport, seriously overestimate how long it will take. Now, double it.

2. Bring an obscene number of snacks and drinks

Partly for bribery, partly to keep your children happy and partly for you to steal off them when you inevitably need some sugar.

3. Make it fun

Our children have always looked forward to appointments because they know they'll get a new colouring book or felt pens. Treat them to something, and don't forget to treat yourself to a new book too. Have a look if there's a nice coffee shop or restaurant nearby that you can go to. After appointments at Great Ormond Street, Zoe loves going to a café in Bloomsbury, while Edward has always enjoyed looking around the LEGO Store in Leicester Square.

4. Expect to be kept waiting

You will be sitting in a waiting room for quite some time, so make peace with it now. Remember to take your new book. Actually, why not take this book? Then you can turn to this page and say to yourself, 'Blimey, he wasn't wrong about the wait!'

5. Try not to move appointments

If you really need to change the time or date, then so be it, but endeavour to avoid this if possible. You're likely to cause yourself so much hassle, I guarantee you'll instantly regret it.

6. Schmooze your consultant's secretary

It's notoriously difficult to get hold of anyone in the NHS, so it's a good idea to find out the name of your specialist's secretary and the direct phone number of the department. We have relied on them for everything from arranging dates for Zoe's operations to little favours such as ordering parts for her hearing aid.

7. Keep all the letters safe

It's worth investing in a plastic folder to safely file all the correspondence. They usually want you to bring your appointment letter, and you don't want to be late due to a last-minute panic over which drawer you've stuffed it into. It's also handy to have everything organised, especially if the paperwork is as voluminous as our children's. Zoe's hospital reports are on a similar scale to the literary archive of a Victorian novelist who lived to 104 and kept copious diaries in an idiosyncratic shorthand.

5

F IS FOR FRIENDSHIPS

Whether you're the parent of a *Coldplay* or a *Zappa*, you'll obviously want your child to have friends. So long as they're a good influence, that is. If we're sticking with musical analogies, no one wants their lovely clean-cut Beatles – all smart suits and happy two-minute pop songs – to fall in with an Indian yoga guru, suddenly grow their hair long, get into drugs and produce anything as horrific as 'Revolution 9'.*

For most mums and dads, their concerns will be limited to who their children are pals with. In contrast, us parents of *Zappas* worry whether our kids will ever form friendships at all. It's truly devastating for anyone to think of their child being lonely and friendless, and heartbreakingly this is the reality for many of us. Children who are a little outside of the norm can often find it challenging to fit in with their peers. Some have

---

* To be clear, this is just an analogy. But genuinely, while I can live with long hair and drugs, I'd be gutted if my children produced anything as embarrassing as 'Revolution 9'.

speech delay and can't easily communicate with their classmates. Some have trouble sharing and taking turns. Some are prone to unpredictable behaviour that can frighten other children. Some don't want to play team games and would rather sit on their own in a corner, obsessively playing with LEGO. And some have the surname Blaker and are likely to do all the above.

In my children's defence, this might have nothing to do with their diagnoses and could simply be genetics, because I wasn't too dissimilar. I had friends growing up, but I was never in the cool gang and rarely played in larger groups. Even as a teenager, I wasn't in any cliques and generally stuck to one or two close friends with whom I could discuss my many obsessions. Football, *Doctor Who*, *Star Wars*, James Bond films, TV comedy shows and American wrestling. And I used to wonder why I wasn't successful with girls.

Given from whose ballsack my boys emanate, perhaps I shouldn't be surprised by their unusual inter-actions with their peers. Indeed Ollie, ostensibly a *Coldplay* and diagnosed with nothing except dumb inso-lence and epic shithousery, has never been one for friends. He's always been perfectly content playing with Adam and concentrating on his hobbies: video games, sleeping and attempting to smell worse than the loos at a music festival.

Yet while I'm willing to entertain the idea that *some* of my children's issues might be inherited, there's no question that those with SEN struggle in this area, and it's something us parents find hugely upsetting. I think a major part of the sadness is the realisation that your child is different. Obviously, some disabilities are apparent from birth, but many are only perceptible when we see our offspring alongside others of the same age. Remember, it was observing Adam at a neighbour's second birthday party that prompted us to finally seek intervention. Looking back now, it was clear he wasn't developing as he should, but we had nothing to compare him with, and so it was easy to miss the significance of his speech and dietary problems.

Adam was well on the way to being diagnosed when he started nursery aged two and a half. On his very first day he gave warning to the other parents as to why they might not want to invite him round for a playdate. Confronted with so many new toys, he ran around like a force of nature, determined to *play* with everything. I italicise the word 'play' because while that's what it was in his mind, to the appalled parents watching it was mostly throwing, hitting and breaking. Momentarily frozen with embarrassment, I failed to jump in as fast as I should have done, and so the nursery was wrecked before Adam had even taken his coat off.

My humiliation was about to deepen because now everyone's eyes were on Adam. They would soon discover that he was totally non-verbal and couldn't respond to anyone's protestations with anything more than a grunt. Some parents gave me looks of pity, but most appeared to be utterly horrified that their precious child was going to be sharing a classroom with this uncontrollable monster. Several mums and dads moved their kids away from him. One mother told her son not to be like that little boy over there. A father tutted. At this point Adam was still undiagnosed, so I wasn't even able to shame anyone by loudly pointing out that our son had a disability. I'd like to think perhaps now people would put two and two together and be more sympathetic, but these were less enlightened times. Either that, or these mums and dads were just colossal dicks.

Given what that first morning was like, you won't be surprised to hear Adam didn't make any friends at nursery. While other little boys and girls chatted at the end of the morning, Adam would be on his own, usually wheeling a toy car on the playmat. Even worse, he was never invited to any birthday parties. Having seen the trail of destruction Adam inflicted on the nursery, parents probably didn't fancy the risk and doubtless thought we wouldn't find out. But when someone let it slip that everyone had enjoyed Johnny's third birthday party, the truth suddenly dawned on me. They'd had a party without us.

Many primary schools have rules about this. If you're going to have a party, everyone must be invited. However, there are loopholes that canny parents can employ. The requirement only applies if you want the staff to distribute the invitations. If it's done by text or WhatsApp, then there's not much the school can do if some children are left out. Nonetheless, parents should think very hard before doing this because realising Adam had been snubbed was crushing. Birthday parties were just one more childhood landmark, along with playdates and first friendships, that were happening without him.

Dear reader, if there's anyone like Adam in your child's class – someone who appears a bit wild or naughty – I beg you, please do everything you can to include them. The fact you aren't aware of a diagnosis is meaningless.

Maybe the parents are still processing that something is awry and haven't yet got the ball rolling. Perhaps the child is still too young to be assessed. It could be they've started on the journey but aren't ready to share this information with you. I appreciate some children's behaviour can be unpredictable. We once had a family round for lunch and, while the parents relaxed, their neurodiverse son proceeded to break our oven. We didn't ever tell his mum and dad, partly because we didn't want to be *those people*, and partly because we're the classic British types who'd rather suffer in silence than face confrontation.* But just because a child is particularly challenging is not sufficient reason to leave them off a birthday party invite list.

There are things you can do to mitigate the risk of your oven – or any other part of your house – being damaged.

- Call the parents. Explain that you really want their child to be at the party, so you'd like to know what you can do to help facilitate this. If you're worried they may be offended, trust me, they'll be more touched by your kindness and understanding.
- Invite the parents to come along. Not in a 'you need to come with and stop your crazy child destroying my house' kind of way. More along the lines of, 'We want your child to be able to enjoy themselves, would it help if you stayed?'

---

* If either half of that couple happen to be reading this and realise who I'm talking about, the repair cost £300, so why not buy twenty more copies of this book as a goodwill gesture?

- Warn the parents ahead of time if there are going to be animals or loud music in case that's going to be problematic for their child. Perhaps you could even offer a separate room in case the entertainer and games get a bit too much. A noisy party with grandparents taking photos and parents fussing over their children can be a sensory overload. A quiet space with a few toy cars or trains would allow the child with SEN to feel included, but with a safety valve in case it starts going wrong.

It may well be that the parents say no. We did on many occasions because we thought it wasn't going to be enjoyable for one of our children. And possibly a few times because it wasn't going to be enjoyable for me. But please, let that be their choice, not yours.

As upsetting as Adam's nonvitation was at the time, it appears even worse when I contrast it to how Zoe was treated at the same age. Before attending a special school, she was in a mainstream nursery for two years and the reactions from other parents couldn't have been more different. It turns out a little girl with Down syndrome is rather more palatable to most people than an autistic boy with a crazy look in his eye. Zoe was cute. At three she was comparable to a baby, still unable to walk, and would crawl across the nursery carpet as if she were an excitable puppy. Like all children with Down syndrome, she had a kindly and sweet face, her tongue usually stuck out of her mouth inquisitively and with a broad smile for anyone that interacted with her. This wasn't a child to be afraid of; this was someone to coo over. But no one ever witnessed Adam running around the playground like a whirling dervish and went, 'Ahhhhh, isn't he lovely.'

It would appear Down syndrome isn't as alarming for other people as autism. Hence, while most children at nursery would give Adam a wide berth, they played with Zoe as though she were a doll. Likewise, mums and dads would encourage their children to involve Zoe as much as possible; a chance for parents to perform some virtue signalling and an opportunity to get their kids doing voluntary work. Never too early to start thinking about their UCAS form. Zoe was also asked to all the birthday parties, though no one ever gave much thought as to how they could meaningfully include her, so we soon stopped accepting these invitations.

I realise this sounds like I'm never happy. Of course, I'm pleased that everyone was so nice to Zoe. It's just a shame that it seems most people are very accepting of children with special needs, but only if they sit quietly, look adorable and never throw toys at anyone. There is also a fundamental difference between autism and more visible disabilities. Anyone can see that Zoe has Down syndrome, so even if her behaviour was more difficult – and believe me, she could be very demanding when it suited her – most people would be sympathetic. Likewise, no one would dare tut or look disapprovingly at a child with cerebral palsy. But children with ASD, ADD, or ADHD generally look like any normal *Coldplay*. Thus, when parents saw Adam they would jump to the worst possible conclusions and think this was simply a naughty boy whose parents couldn't control him. The latter part was possibly true, but the first part definitely wasn't.

There was a period when we were so concerned how people might react to Adam's behaviour that we bought him a T-shirt from the National Autistic Society that read, 'I'm not naughty – I've got autism.'* No parent wants to be shamed by other mums and dads, so this seemed like a good move. However, while I'm sure this top is based on the best of intentions, it wasn't quite the success we'd hoped for. For a start, despite not being able to read, Adam somehow discerned the tone of the message and would act even more outrageously than usual when wearing it. The transformation was so instantaneous that we wondered if the T-shirt had magical powers. Maybe this item of clothing *gave* the wearer autism. It would certainly have been a cunning plan on the part of the National Autistic Society: increase awareness of the charity by selling a T-shirt that not only bears its branding but also multiplies the number of cases. I believe this is what they call 4-D chess.

A bigger issue with the T-shirt was that the crucial line about autism was so small, one would have had to get pretty close to our son to read it. It was certainly nowhere near as large as the name of the sponsors on the football shirt Adam would frequently wear. The irritating upshot was that far fewer people would have been aware Adam had autism than seen his endorsement of Carlsberg. I wouldn't mind, but he hadn't been paid for this and never even received a free bottle.† Nor was the

---

* Turn to 'E is for Embarrassing Photos' to see Adam modelling it on a day trip to Woburn.

† Carlsberg don't do autistic boys, but if they did, they would probably be the best autistic boys in the world.

word 'autism' on the back of the T-shirt, so you literally had to be standing in front of him, no more than five feet away. The only people sufficiently near to see the words tended to be other children, who either couldn't read or didn't know what autism meant. To truly achieve the desired effect, one of us would have had to follow Adam around with a large placard featuring the words 'I'm not naughty – I've got autism' in three-foot lettering and printed on both sides. Don't think we didn't contemplate it.

This being said – and to end the chapter on a more positive note – despite their refusal to conform to normal societal values, our autistic sons have always made friends. At least when they've finished nursery, that is. They've never been the most popular children, but our fears that they might be unable to connect with anyone else were unfounded. Quite the opposite, because in my experience other *Zappas* naturally gravitate towards our kids. In fact, I think their schools now test whether a child has special needs simply by whether they're friends with my boys. If your son is pals with a Blaker, the London Borough of Barnet will give him a personal teaching assistant without even going to tribunal.

This isn't only limited to school. My boys have made instant friendships at soft-play centres and at parks, nearly always with other little boys, usually based on nothing more than running around after each other while screaming at the top of their voices. These crazed games of chase are almost a mating ritual for the autistic child, who can somehow glean everything they need to know about their new friend in much the same way dogs can from sniffing each other's behinds. This is play at its most primal and is perfectly suited to the non-verbal. Grunt, growl, gallop and chuck plastic spheres at each other in the ball pool while all the other children take cover. What more could you want from an afternoon at a soft play? Well, clearly better behaviour if you're the manager, which may explain why we never returned following the nadir which was 'ClownTowngate'.

This stripped-down, basic form of play comes so naturally to my boys, that even when they were finally able to talk, they mostly ignored speech and continued in much the same way. They'd never bother with anything as polite as asking someone's name. No matter how many children are around, they intuitively know which boys are on their wavelength, and will engage in rough and tumble together until someone gets hurt. I've made eye contact with other parents from across a park playground, and while we've not said it out loud, our looks have said, 'I see that your son is autistic too.' If they ever brought back *You Bet!* on ITV, this would be a great challenge: gather a hundred kids in one place and see if my sons can find the other two children with autism in under five minutes. My money would be on them managing it.

There's only one downside to them making friends with other *Zappas*, and that's coming up next ...

6

P IS FOR
PLAYDATES

If you're the parent of a *Zappa* who is yet to start school, I hope I've allayed your fears. I'm confident they'll make friends eventually. The bad news is that I need to warn you about something of which parents of *Coldplays* will be happily unaware: the horrific experience that is the autistic playdate.*

These aren't playdates as you remember them from your youth. Those I enjoyed in the 1980s were effectively a day off for both my friends' parents and my own, as the children minded each other. I recall scampering off upstairs and amusing ourselves with innocent activities like recording our voices on my cassette player – ask your parents – or creating a shop by pricing up all the items in my bedroom, a symptom of growing up in the entrepreneurial culture of Thatcher's Britain. At least my mum provided some vague supervision, albeit from downstairs while she got on with cooking and ironing. I recollect going to my best friend's and his mother basically throw-

---

* NB: The ASD playdate is remarkably similar to both the ADD playdate and ADHD playdate.

ing us out of the house, telling us to play in the street until it was time for lunch (nearly always fish fingers).

If this is what you're expecting of a playdate between two *Zappas*, let me shatter that dream right now. Your children are not going to disappear and amuse themselves, and if they did, it wouldn't be to do anything as charmingly constructive as creating their own shop. On the contrary, the only person making money will be the builder, electrician or plumber you need to pay to rectify the damage.

We've had many of these playdates over the years. Half the time the children sit completely apart, playing with separate toys and barely looking at each other. The rest of the time they're likely to combine their destructive forces like a hurricane tag-teaming with a tsunami. Or, as Edward would no doubt insist, like the first Death Star and the second Death Star. Whatever it's like, after one of these playdates our house is never in the same state of repair. We've had drainpipes broken by boys trying to climb up onto the roof; radiators dismantled by boys who wanted to see how they work; and IKEA furniture disassembled by boys who clearly felt they'd outgrown LEGO and wanted to move on to something bigger. Interestingly, parents have rarely offered to stay. They scarper as soon as possible, dropping their child off with lines like, 'Isaac loves it at your house because you're so relaxed!' When translated this means, 'Isaac loves it at your house because it's even more mental than ours, and by the time I've picked him up your home will look like Dresden in 1945!'

It may be too late for me but at least I can save others. Here, then, is a handy list of ten things you can do to make your playdate go as smoothly as possible.

1. Lower your expectations

Now lower them a bit more. A bit more. Keep going. Down just a little. Up a bit. Down a fraction. Yeah, about there. This is going to be hard work, much harder than your real job. In fact, it will make your real job seem fun. You're not sorting the laundry. You're not catching up with the new series of *Squid Game*. A real-life version of *Squid Game* is happening right now upstairs in your house, so get off the sofa and sort it out. For what it's worth I've never watched *Squid Game*, but I'm aware it's set in a world where children's games turn deadly. I assume the Korean writers must have been a fly on the wall at some of Adam's worst playdates.

2. Less is more

To be clear, what I mean in this case is *less* time results in a *more* successful playdate. I know that's probably obvious, but I felt it necessary to spell it out since I could just as well have made this heading 'Less is less'. As in, less time results in less mess, less money required for structural repairs and less chance of ending the day with a visit to A&E.

You need to think of this like you would a bank job. You've only got a small window before it all goes wrong, which it inevitably will if you dilly-dally. The aim is to get in and out as quickly as possible, and so long as no one tries anything stupid, there hopefully won't be any casualties. Much better for it to go well and for you to plan a follow-up in the future than to be overambitious and left contemplating where you went wrong. To clarify, I've never had any involvement with a bank job, so this is all taken from watching movies and TV shows. Sincere apologies to any real bank robbers reading this who are horrified by my oversimplification of their profession. I'm sure it's more complex than films make it appear.

3. Agree a pick-up time

I cannot stress this one enough. It's all well and good implementing my hard-earned wisdom that less is more, but it's going to be for nothing if your guest's parents aren't on the same page. Make sure you communicate about this, ideally well in advance. Then, if you agreed to an hour – brave, I'd have gone for 30 minutes, but it's your home – you can remind them when dropping off, 'See you at three!'* I'd even remind the parents that they should keep their phones close by, with the ring volume on maximum, just in case you decide to call it quits prematurely. You don't want any of that 'Oh, my phone must have been on silent' nonsense while you're staring down five hours of putting your house straight.

We've learnt this need for clarity the hard way. Maybe we've not been sufficiently clear, perhaps I mumble, but a remarkable number of mums and dads have arrived to collect their children anything from 30 minutes to three

---

* Please only do this if they're dropping off at two. Sorry to keep stating the blindingly obvious but this is vital. You can't have any misunderstandings at this point.

hours late. Of course, this would be rude in any circumstance, but when it comes to the ASD playdate, when
time is of the essence, it's nothing short of a disaster. I
can't help but think some parents have dropped their
child off, and, not believing their luck, taken the opportunity to turn their phones off and go on a shopping trip to
the West End/enjoy an afternoon at a spa/head to bed for
some uninterrupted sexy time. I can't say I blame them,
now I think about it.

(I feel the need to point out that when I say I can't
blame them, I'm joking, and in fact I very much *can*
blame them. We've lived through some terrible playdates
that have fallen apart a full two hours before parents
have returned. And during this time, we've had to deal
not only with our own children, but also a distressed
young guest. No child likes it when they don't know
where their parent is, and a *Zappa* even more so. The
sight of a little boy with SEN staring out the window
wondering when his mum or dad will arrive is genuinely
heartbreaking. So while I'm mainly addressing this list to
the host of the playdate, if your child is invited to one,
please make sure you pick them up at the agreed time!)

4. Better still, ask the parents if they'd like to stay ... possibly

Hmmm. Mixed feelings on this one. There are obvious
pros and some potentially less apparent cons. On the
positive side, you have an extra pair of hands that could
be invaluable when it comes to breaking up trouble and
clearing up the mess. Not only that, but you now have an

adult who knows the other child. They should be well versed in how to negotiate with them and how best to deal with a meltdown. If a parent stays, it also means there's no need to sweat over their return. They're not in bed, they're right here in your house, sharing the pain. You can even change your plans and cut the playdate short if things start to wobble. What's not to like?!

Plenty, as it happens. You need to be aware that some parents will need as much entertaining as their child. I'd go so far as to say, even worse than the late-returning parent is the mum or dad who stays but wants to distract you by sobbing about their child's diagnosis over a cup of tea in the kitchen. Parental support is a significant need for anyone raising a *Zappa*, but as with all things, there's a time and a place. Much better to save it for a coffee morning or Facebook group than when you're preventing us from supervising our children. I've sometimes wondered if this is planned, the parent and child using a classic diversionary tactic to allow as much destruction as possible. 'I'll keep her busy in the kitchen by crying about your IEP; you take their shelves off the wall. You've got half an hour, now go!' This would definitely explain the events of 'Billygate'.*

By all means take the risk – but be firm. Under no circumstances leave the children alone. Never suggest sitting down over a cuppa. If the other parent even looks like they're about to distract you with a sob story, jump in and propose doing this another time when you'll be less preoccupied. And if you really feel the need to give

---

* Named for the piece of furniture that got demolished, not for the child responsible.

them a drink – personally I'd suggest being rude and not offering in case they follow you to the kitchen, but as we've already acknowledged, I'm a curmudgeonly bastard – insist the other parent stay with the kids, because they're two autistic children and it's your house!

5. Plan the playdate to the minute

The second your guest arrives the clock is ticking, and it's a question of keeping things moving before they inevitably go pear-shaped. Make sure you have a plan and don't fall for the classic mistake of trying to wing it. This isn't a time for improvisation. Who do you think you are, Tony Slattery or Mike McShane?! In this scenario even they'd appreciate a script, unless they were being asked to act out a playdate in the style of William Golding.

Whereas a couple of *Coldplays* might be left to their own devices – in some cases quite literally – the autistic playdate requires you to strategise carefully. Come up with a running order of activities and write it down on a piece of paper, ideally no smaller than A4. If you can go to A2 and have it laminated at Ryman's, then all the better. I also suggest using the 24-hour clock to make it sound more like a military operation. This probably won't make the playdate run any smoother, but it will get you in the right frame of mind, especially if you read it out loud to yourself in advance.

- Fourteen hundred hours – Jacob arrives, coat off, get them settled in the playroom.
- Fourteen zero five hours – toy trains.

- Fourteen ten hours – gather up all the toy trains that are now scattered across the playroom and bring out the toy cars.

Feels good, right? You're now Andy McNab, and this operation is going to be a success. Maybe one day you can even write a book about it like he did (or more accurately, like I have).

6. Supervision, supervision, supervision

Remember, if they're in possession of an IEP, the chances are these *Zappas* have a learning support assistant welded to them all day at school. This LSA is now you. So when you supervise this playdate you're doing two people's job at once. Just make sure the teachers' union don't hear about it or there'll be a walkout.

And there will be lots to supervise, whatever form the playing takes. One possibility is that they play individually while sitting as far apart as possible, as though they were a couple going through a particularly acrimonious divorce. In this case your role will be much like that of a judge, deciding on the custody of a hotly contested train from *Thomas and Friends*. When my children had playdates it was always tempting to go for the simplest arrangement and order joint legal custody. However, since one of the parties was my own child I usually found myself favouring them and granting the other party no more than infrequent visitation, permitting them to play with Gordon, James and Percy only under strict supervision. What can I say? I'm no Judge Rinder.

At least this is preferable to the alternative form of play. This is where the pair go off and entertain themselves, and then irreparably damage your belongings, your home or each other, and most likely all three. Clearly this isn't ideal, so the only option is to ensure the children are constantly supervised. You need to be on top of these kids like you're a drill sergeant. 'Trains away, cars out, at the double, now move, move, move!' Anyone gives you shit, they can drop and give you twenty.

And before we move on, let's ensure that we all understand what supervision means. I'm not proposing merely being present in the room, scrolling through Instagram while keeping one eye on the children to ensure nothing illegal takes place. Maybe I've used the wrong word. A better term is probably 'curation', which sounds better anyway, a bit like when dustmen became waste technicians. You need to curate the fuck out of this playdate because they can't, and it won't be pretty if they do. Now we've got that settled, let's skip to what activities to select.

7. Keep it appropriate

If you're also a parent of a *Coldplay*, you may have hosted playdates before and think you're an old hand. So let's start by taking that experience, ripping it up and putting it in the bin. It's worthless. Please never mention it again. Ideas you won't be needing include imaginative play, reciprocity, conversation and board games. Never a bad thing if that means you don't have to endure another round of *Monopoly*. The more ambitious reader might be screaming at this point, 'But if we don't try to get them to share and take turns, how will they ever learn?!' Noble sentiment, but I suggest leaving that to the professionals. I spent over a year taking Adam to LEGO therapy sessions aimed at encouraging social skills, and I've witnessed first-hand that this is no easy task. Trying to bring harmony to a group of uncooperative juveniles is enough to bring anyone to tears. Just ask the last five leaders of the Conservative Party.*

That's what to avoid. What to focus on instead is a little harder because it will depend on the children's interests and age. I'd say you're on safer territory if you stick to toy cars and trains, action figures and dolls, ball games in the garden, LEGO (other brands of building block are available), musical instruments (remember some cotton buds for your ears) and Play-Doh or plasticine (probably unwise to go for anything messier if you value your home). Just remember that sharing might be hard to achieve, so whatever they're supposed to play with, make sure you have at least two of them.† If the highlight of the playdate is going to be a remote-control car, the excitement could quickly turn to rancour if you're expecting someone to sit and watch. If there's a special toy and you only have one, I suggest putting it safely away and avoiding any possibility of a major incident.

The only outstanding issue regarding activities is to ...

---

* Or past three leaders of the Labour Party for that matter

† I say 'at least two', because you'll remember Adam liked to carry around two of everything, one in each hand. Hence, when he had a playdate, we'd ideally have all toys in triplicate.

8. Agree if technology can be used and for how long

I think I've made it clear that there's real potential for the wheels to come off at any moment. With that in mind, if you feel the end is coming sooner than you'd hoped, you'd be forgiven for resorting to the nuclear option and placing the children in front of a screen. We've all done it and there's no shame in buying yourself some time with the aid of CBeebies. When it gets too much, why not allow Justin Fletcher to step in and take some of the load? He's very good at it and doesn't ever moan about looking after our children, probably because he doesn't have any of his own, so he can go home and enjoy the fruits of his labour in peace and quiet. Lucky bastard! Come to think of it, I'm going off Justin. He was awarded an MBE for his TV shows, especially all the work with SEN children on *Something Special*. But we're the ones raising these kids while he's in a TV studio! When I'm changing Zoe's soiled nappies, Justin's probably at home with his feet up, polishing his medal. Quite frankly, if he's getting an MBE, I deserve a life peerage.

Anyway, my new feelings about Justin notwithstanding, technology might be your friend here. However, it would be wrong to assume that other parents will be on the same page as you. One's use of screens seems to be like adherence to COVID protocols. In the pandemic, everyone thought what they did was the gold standard. Anyone who was a bit more careful than you was a germaphobe, Howard Hughes-level lunatic. Meanwhile anyone who did slightly less was a disgrace, had blood on their hands and was personally responsible for any future outbreak. In much the same way, it seems people feel their family's policy regarding TV, iPads and phones is the benchmark. Those that allow more are displaying a level of parenting somewhere between Homer Simpson and the Gallaghers from *Shameless*. Those that are stricter are basically Amish. So before you pick up the remote control, make sure you've had that awkward conversation about screen time.

'*Obviously* it's only as a last resort – it goes without saying!! – but if things aren't going well, and let me stress, *only* if they aren't going well, would it be possible, merely as a card to have up my sleeve in the worst-case scenario, *in extremis*, very much as a desperate remedy, but how would you feel – and again, I must add, only as a final option – how would you feel about letting them watch *Alphablocks*?'

With that many caveats, what fair-minded parent could say no?

If the other parent is fine with technology, be sure to discuss the finer details. Is a Marvel movie or *Star Wars* deemed too violent? Are the lights or loud noises in a particular film likely to upset the child? Is there a time limit on their watching? How about games on the iPad or phone? And is there an objection to more grown-up consoles like the Xbox or PlayStation? Bear in mind, if you're going down the video game route, my earlier point regarding sharing. If you have *FIFA 22* with two controllers, then great, but expecting a child to sit and watch another playing *Candy Crush* on an iPhone is as unwise as any other kind of turn-taking. When it comes to screens, they need to be able to stare at it together. And if it's staring at Justin, then at least he's gone some way towards earning his gong.

9. Other forms of bribery

Speaking as the parent of *Zappas* – and some disobedient *Coldplays* too – I feel the word 'bribery' gets a bad press. It's usually lumped together with the word 'corruption', has its own Act of Parliament in British law, and conjures images of referees receiving wads of cash in a brown paper bag to favour whichever team is playing Liverpool. There's frankly no other logical explanation for some of the decisions we've had this season. But while I can't pretend to have delved too deeply into the Bribery Act 2010, I don't think there's any legislation against the use of certain forms of inducement when it comes to children. And on the ASD playdate, these may be required.

We've already covered screen time, and for sure, this can be used as a bribe to bring law and order to proceedings.* But filed next to technology in the Rolodex of last resorts is the sugary treat. Again, make sure this has been cleared with the other parents, but if it's a possibility, the proverbial carrot of a chocolate bar, ice cream or lolly may be all you need to get a failing playdate back on track. Just whatever you do, when it comes to the carrot, don't offer a carrot. This might work for donkeys, but is never going to work on any children, and definitely not children with SEN if they're anything like mine.

---

* Literally, if you wish to show them *Law & Order*, but I wouldn't recommend it. The reboot is shit.

Vegetables are the enemy, and the fact this one isn't green and tries to fool you by being the same colour as a packet of Reese's Pieces won't help.

A word of warning, though: have your bribes planned well in advance. If it's an episode of *Charlie and Lola*, make sure it's recorded on your Tivo. If it's a Nobbly Bobbly each, make sure you have a packet in the freezer. If it's £20k in used notes, have it in fifties in a paper bag, hidden behind a radiator in the playroom. Only the fool-hardy would offer the bribe of a trip outside to go and buy a treat. Loading the children into the car or attempting to manage them on a walk to the shops is an unnecessary risk. That's before you've even tried to control them inside the newsagent, while they struggle to decide what they'd like. So many pitfalls can be avoided by thinking ahead.

There we have it; we've lowered our expectations, we've agreed a pick-up time, we've got the sign-off for use of screens and even have a bribe or two up our sleeve. There's now only one thing left to do.

10. Move house

This is a good idea in any eventuality. The likelihood is your house is now completely trashed and is going to take so long to put straight, moving home would be a more sensible use of your time. And if by some miracle the playdate went smoothly, you don't want to run the risk of doing it again. What are the chances of a miracle happening in the same place twice? Better to quit while you're ahead, and the best way to ensure the other parent can't foist their child on you is to up sticks and move. Trust me, whatever happens, get straight on to Zoopla and start the whole process again.

7

B IS FOR BATTLES OVER FOOD

Some people are vegetarian; some people are flexitarian; and some people want to really bore you to tears about how they've never felt healthier eating only nuts and tofu. However, nothing compares in terms of complex and limited diets to that of the child with special needs. There is probably no bigger source of stress in our house than food, and it's rare for everyone to be happy at once. The children believe we're trying to make them starve because we've dared to expect them to eat a normal meal. Meanwhile, Gemma and I are living with the horrendous guilt that by giving the kids what they want we're damaging their health.

Our children's diet is so narrow that our weekly visit to the supermarket is preceded by a prayer that some completely new foods have been invented.

Our Father,
who art in the frozen section,
Captain Birdseye be thy name;
thy ready meals come;

thy will be done
in Tesco as it is in Sainsbury's.
Give us this day our daily chicken fillets;
and forgive us our lack of feeding the children
    healthy food
as we forgive people like Jamie Oliver who would
    make us feel guilty;
and lead us not into temptation of trying to feed
    them anything of nutritional value – it's not
    worth the arguments –
but deliver us from tantrums and accusations of
    trying to make them starve.
Amen.

Thus far, our prayers have been in vain. The scientists at Oxford University were able to come up with a vaccine for COVID-19 in well under a year, but sadly no one can formulate a food that will be acceptable to all my kids. This problem is more on the level of Fermat's Last Theorem, and I suspect the Blaker Conundrum could similarly take 358 years to crack. Basically, we're looking for the creation of the taste-free, smell-free and texture-free chicken. If anyone can ever create this, give that person a Nobel Prize immediately. They'd have changed our lives and probably those of many other parents of *Zappas*.

There are children with SEN who have serious dietary and digestive issues, and some need to be fed through tubes. This undoubtedly causes enormous pain and anxiety for their parents. The only saving grace is that at least there can be no debate over meals. For our autistic sons, asking 'What's for supper?' is just a starting point for negotiations. Gemma might make an opening bid of chicken burgers, but it's as likely to be accepted as your first offer on a house. A recent scientific study found that children with autism are five times more likely to have mealtime challenges such as extremely limited food selections and meal-related tantrums. Indeed, Adam's aversion to almost all foodstuffs played a significant role in him getting diagnosed.

Once, in a misguided attempt to empower the children – or more likely out of total desperation – we asked them to each write down or dictate what they'd like to eat. And after we'd managed to decipher the written answers and concluded it would have been easier to get everyone to do this verbally, we were faced with a depressing confirmation of the culinary challenges we faced. (Or more accurately, the culinary challenges Gemma faced, since my cooking talents don't extend beyond putting frozen chicken nuggets and chips into the oven. Which is no great disaster since that is all my kids eat.) What we needed was something white but also coloured; dry but soupy; stringy yet round; and meat but which contains no skin, bones or meat. The last part of which is less problematic than you may think, seeing as McDonald's have been serving meat containing no meat for years. Other requests included pot noodle; pick 'n' mix; pizza with no crusts, tomato, or cheese; and 'no stupid vegetables'. I'm not sure which vegetables aren't stupid but neither of us bothered to find out.

One boy, really looking to take the piss, asked for crispy aromatic duck. Adding further insult to injury, he followed this in parentheses with the instruction, 'Must

be from a restaurant! Do NOT try to make it yourself!'
I'm not sure what was more incredible: this dictionary-definition *chutzpah*, or that he genuinely thought Gemma
might spend her time trying to make him crispy
aromatic duck. As it happens, she's a wonderful cook
and would normally think nothing of spending hours in
the kitchen creating a meal. But even she wouldn't waste
energy making duck with the knowledge that it would
most likely be instantly rejected for containing duck.
Gemma realised long ago that if she wants to cook for
pleasure, she should make the meal and then immedi-ately throw it in the bin, before opening eight packets of
crisps.

Happily, Zoe doesn't have these aversions to food.
However, her learning difficulties do effect an almost
gleeful delight in making our lives as hard as possible.
So, for lunch she wants toast with honey, but then
changes her mind and now wants peanut butter. No,
chocolate spread. No, plain. With crusts; then changes
her mind to no crusts. Cut into squares; no, triangles; no,
polygons; no, dodecahedrons. None of which she eats
because she doesn't eat toast.

Yet the real challenges are with the boys, for whom
food won't even be considered unless it's entirely
processed and artificial. Let me give you a small insight
into the level of alchemy required to create a meal
acceptable to Dylan. First, it needs to be thoroughly
white. If there's a hint of any colour at all – slightly pink,
tiny speck of brown or, worst of all, something green –
that bit must be cut off and destroyed. And I really do
mean white. Not ecru, not vanilla, not eggshell. Ivory?!!
You must be joking. I mean WHITE.

He's equally exacting when it comes to shape. Pasta may be tubes but never twists. Chips must be long and thin and never crinkle-cut or curly. Even frozen dinosaur turkey schnitzel can only be a *Tyrannosaurus rex* and never a *Stegosaurus* or *Triceratops*. It was claimed during the build-up to the Brexit referendum that the EU had legislation banning bendy bananas, but this wasn't actually true. Dylan, on the other hand, has so many rules about the shape of foodstuffs that if we held a referendum about his place in our house, Gemma and I would be tempted to vote Leave.

Similarly, food should be wholly dry, except when it's drenched in tomato ketchup, which must be evenly spread to his exact specification. Don't even think about haphazardly shaking a dollop out of the Heinz bottle. It needs to be a thin layer on top of the meal, a meniscus of ketchup. It goes without saying that the food should also be totally devoid of taste, except for the taste of tomato ketchup. And, of course, every meal should be completely without smell; and before you say, 'Apart from the smell of tomato ketchup,' the demand for odourless cuisine includes the tomato ketchup. We can only hope that he isn't this demanding when it comes to dating, because otherwise he'll be single his whole life. He'd want someone who's one hundred per cent white, just the right shape and with absolutely no taste, which, coincidentally, is also by and large the marital preference of the royal family.

I suppose we should be grateful for small mercies, given that there are some ASD food rituals Dylan doesn't go in for. I have friends whose children refuse to look at a plate with items that touch. They have to get out a ruler at mealtimes and ensure that each sausage is 5mm apart and that the chips are a safe 2cm away, as if they were practising social distancing. I'm not sure whether French fries can catch COVID, but why take the risk?!

Dylan is so difficult that when he was younger he even applied this level of scrutiny to drinks. There was a period when his only words were, 'Want Ribena, no water in my Ribena, just Ribena,' which he'd repeat 20 times a day. He could instantly taste if his squash had too high a ratio of water versus concentrate, and so Gemma and I had to learn to mix the perfect Ribena with the aid of test tubes, a pipette and an Erlenmeyer flask.

On a related note, I'm not sure if this is unique to our house, but all our children seem to be perpetually thirsty. Perhaps this is the result of their reliance on processed food, with its incredibly high salt content. That I can't say – or maybe I'm going to strategically ignore – but what I do know is that if you ever turned off their electronic devices, the only sound in our house would be multiple young voices pleading, 'Can I have a drink? Can I have a drink? Can I have a drink?'

Don't get me wrong. Obviously I don't want my children to dehydrate, but I've no memory of being like this when I was growing up. I drank, of course. I'm alive now, so I must have done. But first, I was happy with tap water, which, crucially, I'd have been able to get myself. And second, I wasn't drinking literally the whole time. The fable goes that if the ravens should ever disappear from the Tower of London, the kingdom will fall. I think my children believe something similar: if there is ever a time they don't have a drink in their hand, the House of Blaker will fall. Or at the very least, they might be slightly thirsty for a bit.

But there's no question that challenging food requirements is something any parents of *Zappas* will recognise. And it's one of the main ways in which we feel different and, sadly, inadequate in comparison with our peers. While other families probably enjoy each other's company during suppertimes where everyone eats the same meal, ours involve six children sitting in front of six different screens, eating six different meals. And still, no one is happy.

Adam is complaining because even though he's been given a Pot Noodle that, as requested, has had anything resembling a vegetable taken away to be shot and buried in a shallow grave, what he wants for dinner is a sherbet dip dab. Dylan is retching on the floor because there's some cucumber on the table, which while not even intended for his mouth, being green is still sufficiently offensive to his exacting taste buds. Edward is happy with his spaghetti but is screaming because the LEGO set he's insisted on building at the table has inevitably smashed into a thousand pieces and fallen into his food, thus creating a Ragu–LEGO fusion. (If LEGO haven't thought of it already, may I suggest a new range? Edible spaghetti-based building blocks that could be marketed as Rago. Any reader who works for either LEGO or Ragu, please be in touch via the publisher.) Meanwhile, The Bailey is screaming for chocolate chips, Zoe is demanding bread sticks and our perpetually angry teenager Ollie is hissing, 'It's Tuesday! I told you I only eat pasta on a Thursday! Why are you trying to make me starve?!'

All this only happens after a complex negotiation over who sits where, which resembles that mental reasoning puzzle about a farmer who must cross a river with a fox, a chicken and a bag of grain. Dylan won't sit next to Adam because he claims he eats too loudly. Edward won't sit near The Bailey because her iPad doesn't leave room for his. Adam won't look at Zoe because he says her eating makes him sick. And no one will sit near Ollie because they're liable to get punched. Me included.

Recently, we had a man round to repair the washing machine, and he looked at our large kitchen table and was taken by the idea of a big family. He glanced almost enviously at me and Gemma before saying, 'Wow, I bet you've had some really great times round this table.' After we briefly exchanged knowing glances, Gemma smiled politely while all I could hear were ghostly echoes of arguments past:

'I only want white food!'

'My LEGO's in my dinner!'

'I want chocolate chips!'

'Breadsticks!'

'Why don't you ever listen?!'

'Make mine again!'

Ah, what happy days!

And if the unpredictable eating habits of *Zappas* weren't stressful enough for their parents, schools heap on the guilt by insisting on issuing a Healthy Eating Policy. I'm convinced they only do this to really fuck with the Blakers. I already felt remorse that my kids are potentially storing up problems like diabetes and obesity. Now I feel even worse for smuggling banned food into school to feed our hungry children. It's not that I want to break the rules, but this is what having a child with SEN does to you. I've had stand-up rows with teachers over whether Pringles qualify as a vegetable.* I've even sent my kids to school with chocolate spread sandwiches and, when questioned, claimed it was Marmite. I always hope no one does that thing you see on TV where detectives put their finger in a bag and then in their mouth to find out if a white powder is in fact drugs. 'Hmmm, as I suspected, it's the devil's tar, Nutella. Book him!' The classic prison escape usually starts with a file hidden inside a cake; our children are more likely to take a cake hidden inside their files. And I know if they get caught, I'll be summoned to school for a *Transition from full-fat Coke to Diet Coke via Coke Zero planning meeting*. And there will be another box of tissues on the table, unless they've also done something good, in which case there will be a plate of biscuits. Which, ironically, are in breach of the school's healthy eating policy.

The bottom line is that parenting *Zappas* is tough going and sometimes we must stop beating ourselves up. Better they eat something than nothing, and if that means the food wouldn't impress Jamie Oliver, well, sorry, Jamie, but I've bigger fish to fry. Probably in batter, in a way of which you wouldn't approve. A few years ago, having abandoned the idea of family trips, we tried to make things more manageable by taking each child in turn for a day out on their own. When I asked Adam where he'd like to go, I suggested a trip to the cinema, shopping mall or bowling alley. His reply was simply, 'Chips.' I'd have taken him round Alton Towers, but for some reason I found myself sitting on a wall overlooking

---

* In case you're unsure, they don't, as the school clarified in a letter to all parents following 'Pringlegate'.

a dual carriageway while he ate soggy, greasy fries. He then washed them down with a fizzy blue energy drink that looked like type 2 diabetes in a bottle and meant he didn't sleep for 48 hours. The National Trust it most certainly wasn't. Incredibly, Adam described this as the second-best day of his life, the best being the day he discovered that Tesco had a deal on Skittles. But you know what? He was happy, he was fed and for once it hadn't involved an enormous argument.

There have been times that I've felt embarrassed or parent-shamed. During the early days of the pandemic when I'd go to the supermarket alone, people got suspicious at the sight of my overloaded shopping trolley. A woman shouted at me, 'Do you really need all those packets of crisps? The shelves are empty due to selfish people like you panic-buying!' I wouldn't have minded, except for while I remember shops running low on bread and pasta I don't recall reading about a national shortage of Monster Munch. But when you have children like ours, sometimes needs must. So, while Gemma and I – well, mainly Gemma – will keep offering a freshly cooked meal and do our best to encourage good dietary habits, there will be days when dinner is processed, artificial and unhealthy, and that's just the way our kids like it.

If you're the parent of a *Zappa* and can relate to any of this, try to keep in mind the following.

1. Please relax

Of course, it's worrying if you think your child isn't eating, but the main thing is whether they're healthy and growing. We had Adam's blood tested to check the level of his nutrients and were amazed to find out they were relatively normal. If he was OK on his diet, your child is probably fine as well!

2. Don't be influenced by peer pressure

Both printed and social media are full of food bloggers and celebrity chefs telling us what our kids should eat. Raising children with SEN is hard enough. Don't let Jamie Oliver and Annabel Karmel's campaigns for nutritious home-cooked food put more pressure on you. Take a step back. Realise, this isn't for everyone.

3. Remember, it's about control

One of the biggest reasons children – especially those with ASD – have issues around food is their desire to have control. So don't enter into a struggle. If they want to live on rice cakes and cereal, so be it. Let them win this one. It will make them happier.

4. Fight less

We wasted a lot of time arguing with our boys over food. The less you fight about this, the quicker it will go away. Don't let eating become yet another battleground.

5. Some people are fussy eaters, and that's fine

There are lots of perfectly healthy and well-functioning adults in the world who are also picky eaters. We don't criticise them – well, not to their face anyway – so why do it to our children? One day they will probably drive their spouse mad, but it won't be your problem anymore!

8

Z IS FOR ZZZZZZZ

Raising children is tiring. People tell you that you'll be exhausted all the time, but it's not until you have a baby of your own that you realise the scale of fatigue that comes with caring for a new-born. However, at least if they're a *Coldplay*, things will improve. They'll get into a routine, start sleeping through the night and eventually head off to nursery or school, and you can get your life back on track. If, on the other hand, you've got a *Zappa*, your tiredness has only just started.

My only advice is to catch up on sleep when you can. If they have a daytime nap, take one yourself. If they go to bed early, do the same. If they're at school and this is one of those rare days when you're not going in yourself for a meeting with the SENDCo, then grab 40 winks on the sofa. Come to think of it, mine are all out the house and Zoe's school has just phoned to cancel the scheduled *We've lost one of the lenses from her glasses emergency meeting* – it turns out she'd hidden it in the sand tray – so apologies, but I'm not going to waste this golden opportunity talking to you. I'm having a lie-down for an hour.

Back soon.

9

I IS FOR IGNORING THE IDIOTS

June 2014
Ext: A park somewhere in north London.

Ashley is sitting on a park bench. He's watching his boys playing while also trying to keep his distance. He's reading a book to make it appear he's someone enjoying the outside rather than the parent of the wild children, or even worse, the kind of man who enjoys staring at other people's kids.

Adam is nine years old, Ollie is eight, Dylan is six and Edward is four. They're running about like crazy animals, which is generally how they played at this age. There are only a few other people around. This park is usually very quiet, which is why Ashley chooses it as a regular destination; he wouldn't want to take his boys where there would be lots of children for Adam and co to terrorise. (Ashley hasn't stopped to consider that this park is so empty *because* he frequently brings his boys here.)

A mother of two sits down on the bench. They smile at each other.

WOMAN: Are those your boys?
ASHLEY: What's that?
WOMAN: The ones over there, pulling each other
by their hair.
ASHLEY: Oh, them? Yes, they're my sons.
WOMAN: Ooh, you've got your hands full.

Ashley gives a half-smile and looks back at his book.

WOMAN: Have they always got this much energy?
ASHLEY: Sorry?
WOMAN: Have your children always got this much
energy?
ASHLEY: Oh yes, 'fraid so.
WOMAN: Wow, you've got real boys.

The End.

This type of scenario has been acted out on many occasions during my time as a parent. I have genuinely heard the phrase 'Wow, you've got real boys' several times, and now realise it's basically a euphemism for 'Keep your wild, feral kids away from my children'.

I'm afraid to say, if you're the parents of a *Zappa* you may need to get used to hearing crap like this. It seems there are many idiots out there who think we want to hear their opinions about our children. Or perhaps they know we don't want to hear their opinions but are such total and utter pricks they demand we listen regardless. I'm not sure which is worse. Either way, you'd better steel yourself as you'll inevitably encounter other people in the playground, in the park, at soft-play centres and family gatherings who'll be only too keen to share their theories about where you're going wrong, how your children could be helped, and how they read an article in the *Daily Mail* that said autism could be cured by cutting out gluten and dairy.

Among the idiots, there are various types to look out for. Here is a brief spotter's guide: what you might have seen had Collins Michelin published a book called *i-SPY Twats*.

1. The Ones Who Think Your Child Just Lacks Discipline

A child with SEN, especially one who has ASD, will often appear to the casual observer as naughty. This is why the National Autistic Society sold that T-shirt: 'I'm Not Naughty – I've Got Autism'. (I like to imagine Nick Robinson wore a similar T-shirt when he took over presenting the BBC's *Today* programme: 'I'm Not Naughtie – I'm Robinson'. And if that's not a dad joke, I don't know what is.)

Now it's one thing for a bystander in the park to think an autistic child is naughty. They don't have access to NHS records, and while one would hope people would give a child the benefit of the doubt, that's not human nature except for the most sainted among us. And to be honest, had Mother Teresa encountered Adam when he was younger, even she would have thought the worst. However, my issue is with the next step in the thought process: that if this child is badly behaved it must be the fault of the parents for not raising them properly and instilling some discipline.

It's this line of reasoning that has led interfering dickheads to utter lines to me like, 'I think you just need to be a bit stricter with your children.' No, you need to be a bit stricter with your mouth and learn when to keep it shut, you complete arsehole.

Some have gone even further and offered to show us how it's done. A parent at the boys' primary school once said, 'Just leave them with me for a day and I'll sort them out for you.' I remember being very torn. Should I tell this person to fuck off, or accept the kind gesture and have my boys destroy their home? The latter was certainly tempting, and I could have given Adam a couple of cans of energy drink to absolutely guarantee the desired result.

Quite why these cretins feel the need to offer their help is beyond me. I can only think it boosts their self-esteem to go around telling people where they went wrong. Why can't they do what I do, which is laugh at other people's mistakes behind their backs? That's much more polite. And don't pick on the disabled! You wouldn't have gone up to the parents of Helen Keller and said, 'Just leave her with me for a few hours; I'll have her seeing and hearing!'

Interestingly, no one ever offers to take Zoe and cure her Down syndrome; but because our boys' disabilities are invisible we get all the bellends who want to volunteer their wisdom. If you truly want to help, be my guest.

I'll drop them round tomorrow morning, and Gemma and I can have a day off.

2. The Non-Believers

We live in a golden age of sceptics who refuse to accept the facts in front of them. They revel in their stupidity, imagining themselves to be rebels who don't uncritically follow what the mainstream media or government tells them. COVID isn't real, climate change is made-up and Trump won the 2020 election. Which is fine, so long as I can believe I've won an Oscar and Liverpool won the quadruple in 2022. But by far the most infuriating of unbelievers are those that deny my children really have special needs.

In many ways *The Non-Believers* are close cousins of *The Ones Who Think Your Child Just Lacks Discipline*. The subtext is the same – that our kids' issues derive from elsewhere – but this group are even more offensive since they deny the reality of our children's diagnoses. The previous group may think behavioural symptoms can be alleviated by a firm hand, but they don't necessarily refute the possibility that their condition is authentic.

Again, in our experience this has related more to the boys. Anyone with working vision can see Zoe has Down syndrome, and it's well established that this is caused by an extra chromosome. There are those with outlandish theories about *why* people might be born with Down syndrome, but even Glenn Hoddle would agree this is a genuine disorder. The more hidden disabilities, though, appear open to debate. Hence, several people have said things to me such as, 'Are you sure this is real? No one had ADHD when we were at school.'

Agghhhhhh!!!!!!! Just because it wasn't diagnosed back then doesn't mean kids didn't have it. You've probably not been diagnosed either, but it's clear you suffer with judgemental-prick-itis. Be careful you don't pass it on to your family.

I'm grateful that we live in an era where our children's conditions are widely recognised and schools are more open to providing help. The comedian John Bishop is dyslexic and has spoken on stage of how different things were when he was young. His teachers told his parents, 'Can you just make sure John can lift heavy stuff?' Unfortunately, the downside is there will always be those that like to play devil's advocate and insist these new-fangled conditions didn't previously exist.

I highly doubt this is you, dear reader, because why would you waste your time on a book about something you think is made-up? I often hate-watch videos on YouTube, but they're usually no more than a couple of minutes long. I possess an incredible amount of spite, yet even I have never hate-read a book, though admittedly I'm a particularly slow reader, so it would be an act of serious sadomasochism. However, on the off chance you're a *Non-Believer*, I'm not going to try to convince you otherwise. What would be the point? All I can ask is that if you ever meet me, Gemma, or any other parents of *Zappas*, please think before you speak. Our children's diagnoses are real, what we deal with is real and the fist you can expect in your face will also be real. Thank you in advance.

3. The Shit for Brains

These are the people who can't resist saying the dumb-est thing possible. They don't have an agenda, so in their favour they're not trying to prove their superior parent-ing skills, nor are they doubting the veracity of your child's condition. To give them the benefit of the doubt, it could be social awkwardness and not knowing how to respond when coming face-to-face with parents of a *Zappa*. Just as people are never sure what to say to a mourner at a funeral or when visiting the terminally ill, I accept it's hard for others to know how to talk to us about our children. But, even with this mitigation, it's still incredible that people come out with the following:

a. 'He's got autism? Really?! He doesn't look autistic.'

And you don't look like an ignorant knob-end but here we are. Let's get this straight: autistic children don't look autistic. They look like children because that's what they are. An autistic child can be white, black, Asian; tall, short, medium height; brunette, blonde, ginger; skinny, chunky, average build; olive-skinned, fair, freckly. Plus every other possible look you could think of. Some behaviours of an autistic child *might* – and I can't stress that word enough – *might* be apparent to the naked eye, but that's by no means a dead cert, or indeed even likely. And what do they think an autistic person looks like anyway? Dustin Hoffman circa 1988? Maybe Maurice Moss in *The IT Crowd*, sitting in front of a computer wear-ing a short-sleeve shirt and tie? Or perhaps they simply expect everyone to wear an 'I'm not naughty – I've got autism' T-shirt? It would at least help *The Shit for Brains* who apparently need a clearer sign.

b. 'Is he high functioning or low functioning?'

Blimey, he's not a television set! There's no sticker on a youngster's back that says how many pixels they contain: 2160p for the 4K, Ultra HD image of an autistic child. (In case you didn't realise, this isn't what's being referred to by the final two letters of ADHD.)

This moronic question is the one I've heard more than the others, probably because it could apply not only to my boys but also to Zoe. In fact, it's regarding her that this has been asked most frequently. People seem to be obsessed with how high functioning she is, as if there were a definitive answer. Of course, there isn't at all. There are actors with Down syndrome who work on TV, and I'd imagine they are more high functioning than others with DS. Likewise, there are those I've seen on *The Undateables* who are not only able to date but can articulate what they're looking for and how love makes them feel. Can I imagine Zoe will be like them? If I'm honest, no I can't, but then she's only 13 and who knows how she will develop over the next decade. For now, I know what she can do, and I know what she can't; I know what I'd like her to be able to do, and I know what it would be unreasonable to expect of her. But none of this can be summed up by either one of the binary options: high or low functioning.

Anyway, regardless of whether there's a definite answer, if you're thinking of asking if a child is high or low functioning, may I suggest you mind your own business? There's a good chap.

c. 'Is your child an artist or musical genius?'

Ugh!! You know, I've come to hate *Rain Man*. It's reinforced this idea that every autistic child has savant syndrome and will be able draw the New York skyline from memory or play any piece of music on the piano by ear. I can't believe I even have to write this, but it's not true. In fact, it's very rare, with somewhere between 0.5 and 10 per cent of those with autism also having some kind of savant ability. So, do me a favour and stop showing your ignorance by asking as if it's a given.

My sons aren't like Raymond Babbitt in *Rain Man*. Nor are they like the kids at Xavier's School for Gifted Youngsters, as much as my Marvel-loving boys would love it to be the case. Dylan is certainly very good at art, as demonstrated by his appearance on the BBC series *Britain's Best Young Artist*. But he didn't win and was beaten by children who, to the best of my knowledge, weren't autistic. Well, they didn't look autistic.* Maybe he'll be able to turn it into a career, which is very much his aim, but it would be stretching things to say he's in any way a savant. He's not producing intricate and highly detailed drawings from memory, apart from reproducing scenes from *The Simpsons*, which he's watched so many times it would worrying if he couldn't draw them without visual reference. Meanwhile, Adam displays no signs of savant syndrome whatsoever, unless you count his

---

* If it wasn't obvious, that was a joke!

remarkable skill to lose his bus pass, start an argument in an empty room and manipulate every single situation to his own advantage. If being shit-hot at those makes you an autistic savant, then yes, Adam pisses on Ray Babbitt from a great height.

And finally:

d. 'I know what you're going through. My sister has a neighbour whose nephew has autism.'

Please, unless you've got a child with autism or [insert name of other disability], you don't know what we're going through. Even if you do have a kid with SEN, the chances are your experiences aren't going to be the same as ours, because every child is different. But at least we'd be able to swap war stories and show empathy for each other. However, if you don't have direct experience, then you really have no idea, even if your sister's neighbour, your brother's boss or your second cousin once removed's gardener has a child with autism.

It's much better to say, 'I don't know what you're going through, but I'm sure it's tough and I'm happy to listen if it would help.' I'd have genuinely appreciated the opportunity to unload had anyone ever offered. And if you're the parent of a *Zappa* and someone asks you to explain the challenges, feel free to save time by purchasing them this book instead. Just don't lend them your copy; this isn't a library. HarperCollins don't print that legal stuff at the front for their own amusement.

4. The Toxic Positivity Dumb Fucks

I need to preface this by saying I'm aware that at this point it looks like I'm never happy. Because just as I get pissed off by those who refuse to believe our children's needs are real, I'm equally if not more agitated by those who go too far in the opposite direction.

There's nothing wrong in having sympathy and understanding. It's great, especially if you give us time to vent and share our feelings. You could even offer some practical assistance, whether with childcare or babysitting, so your friends can have a rare evening off. At least that would be of help. What is of no help whatsoever is coming out with annoyingly mawkish aphorisms such as:

a. 'Everything happens for a reason'

Agreed, the reason being I really wanted to spend the next 15 years enduring interminable NHS clinics; attending speech therapy sessions and school meetings; hosting catastrophic playdates; worrying about my children's eating; and avoiding people like you who will tell me that it's all for the best.

b. 'Having a child with special needs is a gift'

Well, I'm certainly not wishing my kids away and obviously we love them very much. They are a gift, but this is because they're unique individuals, not because they've been born with special needs. This line minimises our experiences as parents and is not what we want to hear, especially if our children have only recently been diagnosed. It might be that with time, parents will reach some level of acceptance and may even view their children's needs as a gift or a means to gain a new perspective on life. But that would be their choice and the result of their personal journey, not because some moron told them to see their children this way.

And worst of all possible toxic positivity is this one:

c. 'God doesn't give you anything you can't handle'

This is genuinely one of the most annoying things one could possibly say to the parent of a child with SEN (or anyone who's dealing with serious illness, unemployment or other form of misfortune). Not only is it unbearably saccharine and incredibly unhelpful, but it also assumes the other person believes in God to begin with. Considering most people in the UK – especially those of child-bearing age – don't believe in God or any higher power, this seems an audacious statement verging on the evangelical. It's tough enough raising a *Zappa*, without anyone using it as an opportunity to convert us. This is a time to offer support, not proselytise.

Even if you know your audience is religious, I guarantee this won't make them feel any better. The implication is we should be able to cope and so if we can't, then it's our failure. If anything, that would make me stop believing rather than putting my faith in a god who wants to test us by making our lives as challenging as possible. What if God gives us things we can't cope with? What do you say to people who are really suffering in life, who have clinical depression or are contemplating suicide? Here's an idea: if you're tempted to voice anything as banal as, 'God doesn't give you anything you can't handle,' shut your mouth and keep it that way.

There is, however, one final group of idiots who to my mind are worse than all the others combined. Forgive my language when I refer to this category as ...

5. The Ultimate Cunts

The reason I give them this epithet is because they know what they're saying, but don't have the bravery to come and say it to your face. There's no pretence of being help-ful or encouraging you with a spiritual message; this is just outright cuntery. What am I referring to? The people I've heard whisper words to the effect of, 'There must be something going on at home.'

Yes, clearly those NHS professionals who diagnosed these children as autistic didn't know what they were talking about and had overlooked the simple fact that our sons had been exposed to some terribly inappropri-ate things on YouTube. Granted, they may have also been exposed to some terribly inappropriate things on YouTube, but that's not the point.

This one really rankles because I've heard it so many times, as I'm sure have other mums and dads of *Zappas*. It's the 'no smoke without fire' take on our parenting. We've all heard the murmurs. All of us whose children have behaved so weirdly, so badly, so crazily that the only seemingly logical conclusion has been that there is something weird, bad or crazy going on at home. It has happened to us countless times, as you can well imagine having read about some of the unsavoury acts perpetrated by my offspring.

So, let me clarify to the billions of you reading this book: special needs children do all manner of potentially embarrassing things. Public swearing, acts of nudity, breaches of various sections of the Public Order Act 1986. And absolutely none of this is indicative of something going on at home. It's indicative of them having special needs. Because to the best of my knowledge neither Gemma nor I have ever wandered around the supermarket shouting profanities; we've never hit our siblings with the first thing that came to hand; and we've never left the house with our genitals on display. All right, once, but I've since thrown those trousers away, and I wrote letters of apology to all our neighbours following 'Tadgergate'.

We speak to each other politely, though sometimes we fight. We're mostly punctual and organised, even though we have the occasional blunder when the wrong child ends up in the wrong place wearing the wrong clothes. We do fun family activities, even though we sometimes use a screen as a babysitter. We shower regularly, pay our taxes and don't jump red lights. During COVID we kept to the guidelines and didn't throw any parties masquerading as a work event. I'd say, by and large, we're decent people. By no means perfect, but definitely respectable. So why do our kids stubbornly refuse to fall into line? Because they're their own people. Parenting them is not a science experiment with a clear cause and effect. Some children, especially those with SEN, will take your noble example and somehow end up with public nudity. If only our teenagers did copy what they saw at home, maybe they'd brush their teeth rather than making Shane MacGowan look like Simon Cowell.

I'll never forget the time that Adam, aged nine, stood in the queue at the Post Office and confidently asked us, 'What does "fuck" mean?' Other people looked on with horror and one woman covered her child's ears. 'Where did you hear that word?' Gemma asked him. He pointed to a man filling in a passport renewal form with the word emblazoned across his T-shirt. We were so delighted at this conclusive evidence that Adam could finally read, we were initially willing to ignore his new interest in swear words. Yet everyone who heard him over the next few weeks would have presumed his new language acquisition was due to something going on at home. 'He saw it on a T-shirt!' we'd vainly protest to his concerned teachers. 'That's what you get for teaching phonics so successfully!' No one was convinced, probably because they knew they hadn't been successful at teaching phonics, and Adam's reading skills owed more to Gemma's hard work outside school hours.*

There's a small minority of cases where issues at home need to be addressed for the physical and emotional safety of children. But for most of us, what is 'going on' at home is nothing more than parents trying, failing, trying again, failing again, and trying one last time, before giving up and letting everyone argue over screens and crisps.

---

* My astute editor has pointed out that this chapter contains so many swear words, any future protestation that our children haven't heard them at home will surely fall on deaf ears.

Much of this chapter has been addressed to the idiots, but beyond a final reminder to keep your mouths shut, there isn't much to add. Instead, let me finish with a message to fellow parents of *Zappas*.

1. You're doing a good job in difficult circumstances

Please remember this and ignore what everyone else has to say.

2. Some non-toxic positivity for you

There may or may not be a God. If there is, He, She, They or It has given you something that you hopefully can but possibly can't cope with. All you can do is try your best and hope it works out in the end.

3. Decide not to take offence

This is easier said than done, considering we live in an age when people are angrier than ever, especially on social media. I'm sure right now someone is tweeting me with a complaint about this book. If it's you, my Twitter handle is @McInTweet. But if we were to get annoyed about every person who says something dumb regarding our children, we'd spend our lives in a perpetual state of fury. If you do encounter these idiots, just remind yourself that everything happens for a reason, and it's

probably a sign of something going on at home. Their
home, which made them such downright twats.

10

G IS FOR GETTING HELP

'Help!'

So sang Bananarama and Lananeeneenoonoo in what is surely the definitive version of this song.* According to interviews, John Lennon wrote it to express his anxiety after the Beatles' quick rise to success, and every day I pray that I too should experience this kind of stress. However, it could just as easily be the anthem for all parents of *Zappas*. Before 2004, I didn't need anyone's help in any way, apart from when it came to putting up IKEA furniture; then I will admit I absolutely needed help from my father. But when Adam was born, those days were gone and I was far from self-assured, although I stopped short at opening up the doors. Adam would have almost certainly run through them and made it down the street before anyone had the chance to come in to provide any assistance.

---

* If you're not aware of this cover, search it up on YouTube. Lananeeneenoonoo were really comedians French and Saunders, and it was produced for Comic Relief. In contrast, the Beatles just pocketed the money from their version for themselves, the greedy bastards.

Almost all mums and dads need help of one kind or another, not least working parents who rely on child-minders to be able to earn a living. But if you have *Coldplays*, it's a much easier proposition. As difficult as it can be to find suitable day care or even a decent babysitter, it all becomes a hell of a lot more challenging if it involves a child with extra needs. Suddenly your options shrink radically. In his early years we couldn't find anyone we felt comfortable leaving in charge of Adam, so Gemma and I barely had an evening out for the best part of a decade. If you wondered why we kept having children, what else was there to do of an evening?!

Even now, we struggle more than we might with finding someone to look after Zoe for an hour before Gemma gets back from work. In truth, nine times out of ten she'd be no problem at all. She comes in from school, puts on her iPad and is happy to entertain herself. It's not like we expect someone to administer a disimpaction or help with a shape test. But hearing that the job would involve caring for a child with Down syndrome is usually sufficient to put candidates off and leave us relying on Adam. Forget the blind leading the blind; the autistic leading the Down syndrome is even further from ideal.

There's just something about the idea of looking after a child with DS that seems to be enough to scare people away. I don't know if it's fear of the unknown or too far from their usual expectations, but that's the way it is. All those ne'er-do-wells in *Scooby-Doo* dressing up as ghosts, witches and zombies to frighten the public away while they hunt for the missing treasure were missing a trick. They should have merely asked people to look after a child with Down syndrome and everyone would have run a mile.*

Even my mum and dad, usually very hands-on grand-parents, appear to be utterly terrified by the prospect of being left alone with Zoe. They regularly take all the chil-dren out for trips or meals and often have them round to their house. They've also kindly had them to stay for a few days so Gemma and I could go away. Considering how houseproud my dad is, and that as little as a stray fingerprint on a window can cause him huge anxiety, it's remarkable that they didn't baulk at entertaining Adam, even when he was at his most uncontrollable. However, for some reason the prospect of looking after Zoe panics them, and they'll do anything to avoid it. They never take her out, and on the occasions Gemma and I have been on short breaks, Zoe has stayed with her former foster-carers Laura and Ian.

For my parents, this was completely normal. On being asked if they'd take the children for a day, my mum once replied, 'Yes, of course, but obviously we can't take Zoe.'

---

* Mention of *Scooby-Doo* reminds me of a one of those stories that only happens when you have non-verbal children. All my boys loved *Scooby-Doo* and in fact still do. Nothing wrong with that, I'm a fan too. Anyway, when Adam was first developing his speech, he knew the episodes by a sound or single word that he could say. His favourite was 'What the Hex Going On?' which, owing to a scary line uttered by the Ghost of Elias Kingston – spoiler alert: he wasn't really a ghost – Adam knew merely as 'Come'. The upshot was that many times he asked me for 'Come'. Even worse, there was an occasion I made the mistake of asking – while in the presence of strangers – what Adam wanted to watch, and he replied simply, 'Come'. If ever there was a time people might have thought there must be something going on at home, then it was this moment, which we now remember as 'Comegate'.

The irony is that Zoe was in many ways the easiest of all the children. Put her on the sofa in front of CBeebies and she'd have sat laughing at *Something Special* and *Balamory* until it was time to go home. Even more ironically, my parents have recently had Zoe along with The Bailey at a time when, being a teenager, she has actually become much harder work than before. Being a dick, I can't resist winding up my parents by talking up the possibility of Zoe's period starting while she's at their house. I know I'm shooting myself in the foot, but I love seeing the look on my father's face as he contemplates the idea of menstrual blood getting on his furniture.

Amazingly, over the years we did find a few brave souls who were willing to do regular childcare, and who even grew to love the children in all their eccentric glory. That said, we had to hunt far and wide, and then lower the bar for acceptability. Our first childminder was Portuguese and barely spoke any English. Beggars can't be choosers, and we thought this shouldn't be an issue when it came to looking after non-verbal children. For the same reason that the largely silent *Mr Bean* was a global phenomenon, I reasoned, Adam could use nothing more than sounds and gestures to exasperate an international audience. Sadly, Julinha was staggeringly unreliable and would often arrive late or not at all, sending a text message at short notice saying, 'My belly ache.' Her stay with us turned out to be similar to her countryman Cristiano Ronaldo's last stint at Manchester United. She cost a fortune, barely ever made an appearance and then buggered off for even more money elsewhere, although thankfully she didn't rubbish me to Piers Morgan on the way out.

Our most recent foray into childcare was a male au pair, the very idea of which freaked people out even more than when we decided to adopt Zoe. Not only that, but Lukas was German, as if with a name like Lukas he could be from anywhere else. On the plus side, his English was better than Julinha's and him being a guy was in many ways a good thing. He couldn't get involved with Zoe's personal care, but he was an energetic older brother to the boys, watching Bundesliga matches with Adam and Ollie, competing with Dylan and Edward at *Mario Kart*, and playing football in the garden in a way I used to be able to before age and crippling athlete's foot caught up with me. It's tempting to also use baldness as an excuse for my lethargy, but it's hardly ever stopped Mo Farah.

Some were also surprised that a Jewish family would have a German au pair, but why not? We never asked him what his great-grandparents were doing in the 1930s and 40s, and it delivered some nice ironies, not least when Lukas would lock himself in his bedroom to avoid having to play more Nintendo with my boys. For once, a German hiding in the attic to escape from Jews, rather than the other way round. Unhappily, it didn't work out in the end. Lukas got very upset when we repeatedly refused to allow his girlfriend to stay, even though we had been explicit from the start that there would be no overnight guests. So we said *auf Wiedersehen* to Lukas and since then, with changes following Brexit, we've had to abandon the idea of having this kind of help. I'm not sure what the rest of Europe thought of the UK for voting leave, but I bet they were at least thankful that now no one would have to move in with the Blakers.

Many parents can rely on friends for occasional help but, as previously mentioned, the trials of looking after Adam caused us to retreat somewhat.* We'd recently moved to a new part of London and had hoped that we'd meet other locals with whom to socialise. Yet we quickly realised that accepting invitations or having guests in our home was not only stressful for us, but also unfair on Adam, putting him in situations that weren't suitable for him to be himself. I've often wondered how different our lives would be if he'd been our second or third child. If, rather than having an often uncontrollable, energetic little boy, we'd had a docile *Coldplay* with whom we could have socialised and forged the kind of bonds we now lack. I imagine it would have changed everything because Adam, bless him, set the tone in our house. All our expectations for what our children should and shouldn't do were established through raising him, and it's undoubtedly made us different parents than we might have been. But as the phrase goes, 'If my aunt had balls, she'd be my uncle,' so it's probably best to leave the what ifs there and move on.†

While not a practical help, Gemma was at least able to get emotional support from friends she met at a group for mothers of children with SEN, run by a local charity. She has described this weekly gathering as a life saver:

---

* For those pointing the finger at me for our lack of friends, I refer the honourable member to the reply I gave some chapters ago.

† I love this saying which, funnily enough, I first heard from my uncle. It is admittedly rather anachronistic and should now be rephrased as, 'If my aunt had balls, she'd be free to identify in whatever way she liked, and apologies to my aunt for using the feminine pronoun, which should be entirely my aunt's choice.'

90 minutes during which the non-school-age children were cared for by volunteers, while the mothers were able to offer advice, vent and listen to each other in a non-judgemental space. She's still in contact with most of these mums and they've shared many of their *Zappas'* highs and lows over the years. Unfortunately, the sporadic attempts to do something similar for the dads always fell through for one reason or another. Being paranoid, I'm now wondering if the many excuses were true, and they were all meeting without me. If this is the case, I still deny it's because I'm a curmudgeonly bastard and is most probably antisemitism.*

It was via the mothers in Gemma's group that we found out about many other resources open to us as parents of *Zappas*. One was a charity that provides horse-riding opportunities for children with SEN. It wouldn't be the world of special needs if this didn't have its own fancy abbreviation, and in this case there are competing versions. It's sometimes called equine facilitated education and therapy (EFET) but also goes by the name equine assisted therapy. Seeing that this spells out EAT in connection with horses, I presume this name is more common in France. Adam did this several times and absolutely loved both the riding and the grooming of the horses. Unfortunately, he has since grown into a six-foot strapping young man, so my hope that he could be the new Frankie Dettori have come to nothing.

Another wonderful amenity we discovered was the Thames Valley Adventure Playground, widely known as

---

* The fact that the group was run by a Jewish charity makes this unlikely but I can't rule it out.

TVAP. I really wasn't exaggerating when I said this world is full of abbreviations. Considering our trips to regular parks and soft plays would usually lead to a riches of embarrassment, outings to TVAP have been the most welcome break from the norm. It is a large, fully enclosed facility near Maidenhead especially designed for children with SEN, and being surrounded exclusively by parents with similar kids is such a refreshing experience. This is a totally non-judgemental space, and it's no exaggeration to say we've never felt more relaxed on days out than at TVAP. During a visit a few years ago someone accidentally took Gemma's handbag containing our car keys and leaving us stranded. When they were returned a couple of hours later, we were sad that we wouldn't be forced to stay and had to go home after all.

Meanwhile, for *Zappas* like mine, TVAP is like Disney World and Disneyland combined. It has huge outdoor spaces in which they can run wild; it's near a lake so they can watch boats; near a train line so they can watch trains; it's filled with everything they like including zip wires, go-karts, swings, mock forts, dress-up, a sensory room, a ball pool and a bouncy castle; plus, there are lots of other *Zappas* with whom they can make friends and chase after. Even better, siblings are welcomed and so it has become an annual trip for the whole family. I think this may be the one time our *Coldplays* have felt privileged to have siblings with SEN and so gain access to the forbidden city. I don't know how many similar places there are in the UK, but if I were prime minister I'd build one in every town and then move in.

Another crucial resource we've come to rely on is a respite charity called KEF (which stands for Kids Have

Endless Fun, as if you hadn't guessed that already). They run a weekly Sunday club that Zoe attends, and twice-yearly residential programmes – a week in the Christmas holidays and a fortnight in the summer – that are unquestionably the highlights of Zoe's year. Three weeks of non-stop activities and one-on-one attention. Dare I say it, these camps are also a highlight of Gemma's and my year: three weeks' relief from caring for Zoe in the knowledge that she's having the time of her life. That said, these kinds of break aren't suitable for every *Zappa*. Both Adam and Dylan have previously been on the summer scheme, and in the latter's case it was more trouble than it was worth. This isn't to suggest he didn't enjoy it. On the contrary, he absolutely loved it. He was given a dedicated surrogate big brother to play with, and this one spoke perfect English and didn't have a natural proclivity for *Lederhosen*. However, while Zoe was capable of having a fabulous time at KEF and then coming back to reality, Dylan couldn't cope with the readjustment. He went twice and on both occasions it was two weeks away followed by four weeks in bed crying his eyes out while clutching his book of camp photos. 'I don't want to be home,' he'd sob. 'I want to be with all my friends and counsellors and do fun stuff every day and not have to go back to school. Why can't every day be like camp?'

It was both wonderful and sad. Wonderful that for a fortnight Dylan had enjoyed something he wasn't accustomed to during the rest of the year: an all-encompassing acceptance and celebration of who he is, an experience that can be rare for a child with special needs. Yet it was sad to see Dylan lose his innocence and discover a fact that Zoe, bless her, may never have the understanding to appreciate: that sometimes life can be a bit shit. Yes, you can have an amazing holiday, but then it's time to return and go back to work. If that weren't the case, half the country would currently be in Ibiza. And so reluctantly, Gemma and I decided we couldn't go through this a third time, and fortunately Dylan seems to have forgotten he ever went away with KEF.

Besides, there have been much more important forms of help required when it comes to Dylan. Like Adam before him, he's a veteran of many a speech therapy session. I am still not one hundred per cent sure how successful they've been. Obviously in one sense they were a triumph in so far as he can now speak, but had we known the monotonous gibberish he would come out with we may have given speech therapy a miss.

'Tell me, Dylan, what did you have for lunch today?' I asked my then ten-year-old son on the way home from school, partly to make conversation, partly to stop him launching into another monologue about something he'd seen on YouTube.

'I'm not sure what you call it. It was green. And spiky. Kinda with holes in it.'

'Green?! Did you like it?'

'Yes. Or maybe no. Come to think of it, maybe it was orange. But it had spots all over.'

When I got home I checked the school menu. The lunch that day was chicken.

If I took Dylan's speech therapists to task over this, they'd no doubt argue their job was to help this boy talk. What came out of his mouth thereafter wasn't their responsibility, and more to do with the unusual thought patterns in Dylan's autistic brain. And while this might be true, I'd still point the finger at them for introducing him to certain expressions and concepts.

For instance, one block focused on teaching conversational phrases, which led Dylan to labour under the impression that 'Don't take this personally' operates as a general get-out-of-jail-free card for saying anything that pops into your head. On the following day alone, we had both a crying teaching assistant and an irate mother on the phone complaining about things Dylan had said along with the caveat, 'Don't take this personally.' Nor was Gemma too impressed when Dylan said, 'Don't take this personally, but your supper was so disgusting that I couldn't even get the cat to eat it. Can I have a sandwich?' I was very tempted to call the speech therapist to say, 'Don't take this personally, but why don't you fuck off?'*

Admittedly, there were times that Dylan would seek me out to engage in conversation, which suggested some progress. 'How are you, Dad? How was your day?'

It would probably have been quicker at this point to simply hand over the £10 that was typically the true intention behind these attempts at civility. For some masochistic reason I liked to delay the inevitable, so I'd try to have some appallingly stilted social interaction for a few minutes before having to cough up. 'Fine, thanks, how are you?' I'd respond.

By now, Dylan would usually be busy with his phone and not answer. Evidently the speech therapist had

---

* I probably would have done if it was my cooking he was insulting, but seeing as it was Gemma's I felt as though I didn't have a dog in the fight. And if you're reading this, Gemma, please don't take that personally.

covered 'Beginning a conversation', but never got on to 'What to do when the victim of your social intent actually answers'.

On other occasions Dylan would just parrot phrases he'd been taught in speech therapy regardless of whether they fitted the context. It was as if he'd been using one of those tapes we listened to in French lessons in the 1980s that encouraged us to *Écoutez et répétez*. The difference is that while I never found any situation when it was appropriate to use *Où est la gare, s'il vous plait?* Dylan didn't let lack of suitability stop him.

'Dylan, why the hell have you squirted shower gel everywhere?!' I shouted at him on finding the mess in the family bathroom.

He looked sheepish, and then a thought almost visibly popped into his head. He gave a half-smile and looked me in the eye. 'I'm really sorry, madam, but I did not understand what you just said. Please could you repeat it?'

'What? You heard me. Why is there shower gel everywhere? And why are you calling me madam?!'

'I am really sorry, madam, but I did not understand what you just said. Please could you repeat it?'

It then dawned on me where this came from. 'Dylan, did they teach you this in speech therapy?'

He nodded.

'Do you know what it means?'

'No, I've got absolutely no clue.'

By this time I could have cleaned up the shower gel myself, but I felt I had to make him realise how annoyed I was at the state of the bathroom. 'Dylan, it's important to be able to read other people's emotions. Look at my face and tell me how you think I'm feeling at the moment.' I screwed up my face into the best and most exaggerated approximation of anger I could muster. 'What do you think, Dylan?'

He thought about it for a second. 'Like you're desperate for a wee?'

'No.'

'Happy?'

My face was beginning to hurt. 'Give it one more go.'

'I am really sorry, madam, but I did not understand what you just said. Please could you repeat it?'

Dylan's speech therapy did eventually cover emotions, but even that wasn't quite the success we might have desired. I once overheard him saying to Edward, 'Feelings are things that speech therapists have. And girls.' Edward nodded along at Dylan's wisdom as his older brother continued. 'You can ignore them, but if someone says you've hurt their feelings you've got to apologise even though there's no blood.' Oh well, you can't say we didn't try.

Despite all this, I'd still suggest that getting assistance from professionals has been completely life-changing for our children. Not only do we have sons who can now speak – gibberish and swearing though it may be – we've also received the ultimate help: medication. I'm sure other parents will have their own view on this subject, but I can only tell you about our experiences with both Adam and Dylan, which have convinced me Richard Ashcroft from the Verve was wrong, because the drugs do work.

I won't dwell on this, as clearly it's something one must discuss with a doctor or psychiatrist. I have no medical training and can't even fix a fungal foot problem. All I will say is that there was Adam before drugs and Adam after drugs, and it's no exaggeration to say that they were like two different children. He benefited enormously as the pills calmed him down dramatically and helped him to concentrate. He was still the same loveable rascal, but it took the volume down from ten to a more palatable six or seven. And if I ever had doubts that the prescription was necessary, when we forgot to check Adam had taken them we'd get urgent calls from his LSA begging us to drive back to school with the meds. When I'd arrive, I'd see a mix of terror and relief in her eyes, the positive impact of the drugs having clearly caused her to forget what it was like to deal with Adam in his natural state. It struck me then that if we ever wanted to get the school to do something, there'd be no better way than threatening to send in Adam unmedicated.

If you do go down the drugs route, all I'll say is that it won't fix everything. After several years of taking his pills with favourable results, Adam became noticeably ruder and more aggressive. We immediately emailed his psychiatrist: 'WE NEED MORE MEDS NOW!!! UP THE DOSE!!! DO SOMETHING! ANYTHING!' This plea was followed by a list of all Adam's recent misdemeanours, organised in 73 bullet points. I hoped these would seal the deal but, alas, they had the opposite effect. The next day the psychiatrist emailed back.

Dear Mr and Mrs Blaker, I'm afraid what you are describing is normal adolescent behaviour. There is no medication for this. If there were, I would have used it on my own kids.

All right then, Richard Ashcroft, let's compromise. The Drugs Don't Always Work. For some problems, you must wait it out.

I know you'll be itching to start researching medication, but before we move on, here are some ideas for how to maximise help for you and the *Zappa* in your life.

1. Keep it formal, even with family

If you can get assistance from grandparents and siblings that's great, but it will make a real difference if you've got an arrangement that you can count on regularly without having to request it each time. You won't be so guilt-ridden about continually asking, and it will hopefully stop them feeling put upon if they know it's only one day a week or once a fortnight.

2. Get on social media

Apologies if I'm stating the obvious, but there are many Facebook communities for parents of *Zappas*. Even if you can't get to the kind of in-person gathering that Gemma attended, you can still meet other mums and dads online and hear about potential resources. Why don't you look for some groups now and post the comment 'Ashley Blaker suggested I join in his amazingly helpful (and also incredibly funny) book!!!'?*

---

* I'd be equally happy with 'incredibly funny (and also amazingly helpful) book'. I'll leave it to you which one to go with.

3. Learn to help yourself

Every parent needs a break, and those with *Zappas* even more so. Identify some small, relatively inexpensive things you can look forward to each week. Put them in your diary and commit to them. Just be sure to have compassion for yourself. You're going to lose it sometimes because we all do. This isn't easy.

4. Set aside time for your *Coldplays*

If you have other kids, then it's important to spend respite time with them. When Adam, Dylan and Zoe went away for the summer, it was very tempting to use the two weeks to catch up on sleep. Instead, we'd spend it entertaining the remaining children with trips, takeaways, shows, picnics and beaches, all of which helped give them the attention they'd often miss out on. Naturally, after a couple of days listening non-stop to The Bailey, we'd be counting down until the others returned and we could get back to our version of normal.

5. Get a therapy dog

I've heard many good things about therapy dogs, but I'll be honest and say we've not had one ourselves. We did sign up for the waiting list, having reluctantly accepted that after 13 years of attempting to teach our boys social skills, a dog could do a better job than me and Gemma.

In our defence, the dog wouldn't also be thinking about clearing the house, cooking meals or when Liverpool will finally win the league. However, in the end, we got sick of waiting and got a cat instead.

6. If all else fails, buy a games console

It's the nuclear option but it worked with my boys. Buy them an Xbox, Nintendo or PlayStation, install it in their bedroom and then leave them to it. All you need do is fling in a pizza or burger every couple of days, and your parenting responsibilities are over until they turn 21.

11

Y IS FOR YOUR SMELL IS TOO LOUD FOR MY EYES

The title of this chapter sounds like a joke, but I can't take credit for this one, I'm afraid. Not that that's stopped me before, but in this case I'll acknowledge the source. This line was uttered by Dylan, although I honestly can't remember which of his siblings he was finding objectionable at the time. The smart money would be on Ollie during his teenage B.O. phase, but it's not important. Just so long as it wasn't me, because I try to stay as odourless as possible.

Before we go any further, let's clarify something right at the top of this chapter. Although sensory issues are common among those with ASD and can themselves lead to a diagnosis, not all children with these sensitivities have autism. Likewise, not all children with autism have sensory issues. And even if a child does have sensory challenges, there's a huge range of ways in which it might affect them. They might have hypersensitivity, which leads to an aversion to certain sights, sounds, smells, tastes and textures, or potentially all the above. On the other hand, they might have the reverse problem –

hyposensitivity – which causes an under-responsiveness to these stimuli. This sometimes leads to children trying to stimulate their own senses by making loud noises, touching things or rocking back and forth.

Happily for this book, though less so for me and Gemma, between them the Blaker children seem to cover every variation of SPD (which isn't a political party but stands for sensory processing disorder, yet another abbreviation for our collection). Dylan is typically untyp- ical – or is that untypically typical? – when it comes to his sensory problems. He can't even eat Coco Pops because he insists they're too loud. A few years ago he genuinely asked me to sift through the bowl and remove the noisiest offenders. Looking back now, I'm wondering if he was trolling me or covertly filming this for his secret YouTube channel: 'Dumb Father Tries to Select Loudest Coco Pops from the Cereal Bowl' – 1.7 million views. I'm inclined to think the best of him and assume this was a sincere request born of his dislike for certain sounds. Anyway, I've always wanted a video of me to go viral, so I'm happy either way. Just thank God we never bought Rice Krispies, because with their tendency to snap, crackle and pop, I'd have spent all day and night searching through the cereal box trying to find the sole noiseless krispie.

And yet, for all Dylan's intolerance of rice-based sounds, I once caught him sitting quietly with a big smile on his face holding an alarm clock against his ear. When I asked what he was doing, he explained that the ticking sound made him feel good. Each to their own. It's a lot cheaper than drugs and is unlikely to be a gateway to bigger thrills. I can't imagine in five years, when the hit of the clock wears off, that he'll be scaling the Houses of Parliament to press his ear against Big Ben.

Apparently, this behaviour is called stimming – short for self-stimulating – and is common among autistic people as a means to preserve balance in their sensory systems. It might be holding a clock to the ear to enjoy the constant ticking, but could equally involve employing repetitive movements, sounds or fidgeting to stay calm and block out any uncomfortable sensory inputs. In some cases, these practices are self-discovered, but Dylan had a dealer of sorts who introduced him to his drug of choice. His Pablo Escobar was Mrs Daniels from his primary school, who had on her desk a Newton's cradle. She correctly guessed that the clicking sound of the balls swinging back and forth would help him to concentrate and learn better. Dylan, however, kept this information to himself and didn't come home asking us to buy him his own Newton's cradle. Which is surprising, since every other day he comes home and asks us to buy him something. If it had been called the Nintendo Newton's Cradle, I'm sure he would have, but he didn't and instead, to his great credit, used his ingenuity to look around the house for something that would replicate the sound.

On hearing this story, Ollie mockingly asked, 'Will buying a Newton's cradle make Dylan normal?' I should have immediately rebuked my second son for his lack of compassion and for implying Dylan was in any way abnormal. I ought to have sat Ollie down and explained that Dylan is perfect just the way he's been made, and that he doesn't need to be anything other than himself. And I did do that eventually, but only after going onto Amazon and buying two Newton's cradles.

It could be that as well as having Down syndrome, Zoe is also on the autism spectrum. Some research suggests around 15 to 20 per cent of people with DS also have ASD. At the very least she clearly has SPD, and will get very distressed by noise, often crying if the TV is on too loud or if me and the boys get too animated when Liverpool score a goal. There was an all-too-brief moment on the last day of the Premier League season in 2022 when Manchester City were losing 2–0 at home, and I became a little over-excited at the possibility of Liverpool snatching the title. This involved me screaming my head off, my face contorted like a living Hieronymus Bosch painting, which caused Zoe to immediately burst into hysterical tears and Gemma having to calm her down. I felt terrible, of course, not least because City came back to win 3–2, and all the celebrating had been for nothing.

The thing that's most strange about Zoe's sensory issues around sound is that she's supposed to be deaf! I've spent hours at Great Ormond Street Hospital seeing consultants about her hearing loss. I've watched her sit in a room as animal noises are played from all directions, while the audiologists monitor her reactions from the other side of a window. We even had a summer ruined by an operation to insert magnets in her skull to allow for bone conduction hearing aids to be placed on her head. (After all the palaver, and having caused a horrible infection on the right side of her scalp that still hasn't cleared up, the specialist helpfully told us she only needs to wear the hearing aid for her left ear. Thanks a lot.)

Given all this, I've always been baffled by how incredibly sensitive Zoe is to any sound. I can whisper something to Gemma in the kitchen while Zoe is watching her iPad in the living room, and she'll still shout, 'Too loud!' I did once ask the consultant if he could explain why he maintains Zoe has such bad hearing loss when I feel it's almost bat-like. He gave a long-winded reply that boiled down to, she hears one kind of sound but not another. He's the expert about this kind of thing, not me, so who am I to argue? Then again, I'm not the one who inserted a magnet behind her right ear unnecessarily.

Meanwhile, Adam's sensory issues make both Dylan and Zoe appear very easy-going. In his younger years Adam's SPD would cause him to get upset about all manner of sensory inputs. And frustratingly, while he knew what it was that troubled him, he often struggled to articulate it. Once he'd learnt to talk, he would come out with all kinds of complaints.

'The popcorn's too bright!'

'These flowers are too spicy!'

'Ollie's breathing my air!'

'Tell Bailey to shut up! Her voice smells.'

At the time, that last one sounded particularly ridiculous, but I could imagine Simon Cowell using this line to put down a wannabe singer on *Britain's Got Talent*.

In his first 18 years Adam has only been to the cinema twice. Lovers of trivia will want to know that it was *Spider-Man: Into the Spider-Verse* and *No Time to Die*, so at least he saw movies with an average Tomatometer score of 90 per cent on Rotten Tomatoes. If you're merely going to go to a couple of films in nearly two decades, you may as well see something decent. However, movie buffs will have already noted these films were released in 2018 and 2021 respectively, which means he waited until he was 14 to even find out that the cinema wasn't for him. Such was his own self-awareness when it came to his SPD, Adam always said no when we gave him the opportunity to come with his siblings to see everything from *Paddington* and *Despicable Me* to *The Avengers* and *Batman v Superman*. And regarding that last film, he definitely made a good call. As it happens, Adam enjoyed watching all these films on the TV – well, not *Batman v Superman*, that was clearly shit – but he knew without even experiencing it that the combination of a dark room, a big, bright screen and stentorian Dolby Cinema speakers would be a bad idea. And that's before we even get onto the sound of loud popcorn consumption, which is enough to drive me mad, so God knows what it would do to someone with SPD.

Another bone of contention for Adam has been clothes. Even now, he's liable to leave the house on the coldest day of the year in a T-shirt and shorts. I'm sure part of this is down to good old Blaker belligerence, but it's mostly because these are among the very few clothes that make Adam comfortable. From a very early age we struggled to find anything for him to wear. Everything was either too tight, too itchy, too scratchy, too heavy, too twisty, too sticky, too wriggly or even too salty. I had no idea how clothes could be too salty, but I knew Adam well enough to accept that it wasn't worth fighting over because he wasn't going to be persuaded.

A major sticking point has always been long sleeves. Adam absolutely refuses to wear anything but short sleeves, no matter the weather, and that's just the way it is. I think this is one case where you can see at once both his hypersensitivity, in that he doesn't like the feeling of material on his arms; and his hyposensitivity, because he doesn't seem to feel the cold. Forget departing a random person's home after a one-night stand, there's no walk of shame to match leaving the playground after dropping off your son who's wearing nothing but a short-sleeve shirt on a freezing January morning. I'd always look down at the ground and avoid all eye contact, but I could almost feel the disapproving stares from other parents. I couldn't face them; their looks were, well, too spicy.

Sometimes the headteacher would catch me before I could make my escape. 'Mr Blaker, Adam really does need to be wearing a coat,' he'd say, perfectly reasonably. I felt so embarrassed. He had a coat; he had a jumper; he had me and Gemma flapping around him every morning telling him to put them on. But he just didn't feel the need, and none of me, Gemma, the headteacher or Tomasz Schafernaker predicting a new ice age on the BBC were going to cut any ice, crap pun intended.

But you know what, we'd done our job. We'd provided the requisite layers and the guidance that he'd freeze if he didn't put them on. We'd fulfilled our side of the parenting bargain; however, Adam wasn't cold, so he wasn't going to come to the negotiating table. It was his life. We just had to let him do what felt right for him, no matter how mortifying it was in front of the other parents, whose kids were all wearing colour-coordinated hat and glove sets. If that makes us sound ultra-permissive then so be it, but I really don't think we are. We don't allow our children to do anything they like while we relax on the sofa watching TV. True, I sometime leave Gemma to parent while I relax on the sofa watching TV, but that's a different thing altogether.

I think I can speak for both of us when I say that we view our job as parents as having two key aspects.

A. To love our children unconditionally.

B. To keep them safe.

If our children want to do things and it's safe, by and large, we let them. It's not ideal to be playing outside in short sleeves, but we knew he'd be running around working up a sweat, and if he told us he didn't feel the cold, we had to believe him.

I'll admit that this second part of my parenting manifesto has been severely put to the test by Adam's SPD. As with many children who are under-sensitive he'd seek out thrills, and he spent much of his youth climbing great heights and then jumping off. We were always the least popular people any time we visited a soft-play centre. Adam would immediately find the ball pool and, with no concern for his own safety and even less for the safety of others, start auditioning for a future role as a stunt man in the Bond films.

In 2009, when Adam was five years old, we took him to Trafalgar Square. Being a large space free from cars it's a great place to take kids, and they can run around and frighten the pigeons instead of other children. That said, I'm sure there will have been some young pigeons on the spectrum who naturally gravitated towards Adam, while older pigeons looked on disapprovingly, cooing to their friends, 'Wow, those humans have real boys!' And they'd have had a point, because at one moment I turned around to talk to Gemma and when I looked back Adam had somehow climbed halfway up Nelson's Column. To this day, I've no idea how he managed this. He was mostly non-verbal at the time, so couldn't properly answer the question himself.

Two years later we took all our children to Berkhamsted Castle. We sat and had a picnic on the grass while Adam and Ollie ran around the ruins of the external wall. Adam even climbed up and down the wall, and everyone had a good day out. It was only when I got home and looked at my photos that I realised quite how far up the wall he'd managed to get.* We immediately signed him up for a session at a climbing wall, deciding that at least there he could get these thrills while wearing a helmet and harness. Inevitably, he loved the climbing, but said that the protective gear was too itchy, so we didn't go again.

Without doubt, the most extreme example of Adam's SPD putting him in danger was from the summer of 2018. It was an incident that has a firm place in Blaker family folklore, although there's some debate about whether it should be known as 'Parkgate' or 'Footgate'.† We had taken our now six children – what were we thinking?! – to Victoria Park in Hackney, east London. At one point, Adam and Dylan went together to play near a shallow pond, while Gemma and I stayed with the others. Adam was 14 at the time and although not the mature young man he is now, we felt he was sufficiently sensible to be allowed to wander off with his younger brother. About half an hour later, the ten-year-old Dylan ran back.

'You've got to come. The park man wants my parents.'

---

* Turn to 'E is for Embarrassing Photos' to see the picture for yourself.

† If you're interested, 'Footgate' won.

'What are you talking about? What park man?' I asked.

'The park man. He said Adam's trainer is red.'

'Adam's trainer is red? No it's not, it's white.'

'His trainer's red.'

'Gemma, what colour are Adam's trainers?'

Gemma looked over nonchalantly. 'They're white.'

'See, Dylan. I told you they were white.'

'No, his trainer used to be white but now it's red. The park man said his foot is falling off.'

I still had no idea what Dylan was talking about. Who was the park man? And why was Adam's trainer now red? There was nothing else for it but to go and investigate.

As we approached the pond I could see a small crowd had gathered. Then, as I got nearer, I could see they were all looking at Adam, who was sitting on the ground with one of the Victoria Park staff beside him. My first thought was that Adam must be in trouble. I presumed he'd hurt another child or perpetrated an act of vandalism. However, once I reached him I saw that his left shoe was indeed red, because it was clearly covered in blood.

What it seems had happened was that Adam had decided to play in the pond, or more specifically jumped right into it. And in a scene that could have stepped right out of one of those terrifying 1970s public information films, he'd landed directly onto a discarded bottle, the glass piercing his shoe and entering the sole of his foot. Due to Adam's SPD, what would have instantly paralysed some people didn't bother him at all. He'd kept playing until the 'park man' saw him and demanded Dylan find their parents. And for his part, Dylan, being Dylan, hadn't put two and two together, and failed to realise there was anything in the slightest bit strange about Adam's previously white trainer having miraculously turned red.

And here we witnessed both the negative and positive sides of Adam's SPD. Yes, it had led to him doing something stupid and then walking around making it worse. But on the other hand, his sensory issues meant that he was spared what should have been unbearable pain. An ambulance soon arrived to take me and Adam to the hospital, and when we arrived at A&E, a doctor took off the now bright red Adidas and I saw that Adam's heel was all but falling off. And still Adam didn't seem too fussed. 'Do you have Wi-Fi here, doctor?' was all he had to say.

The doctor was genuinely baffled, saying that this child should be in agony. He wasn't, he was just fiddling with his phone. She told me she'd normally use a general anaesthetic, but in this case Adam seemed so blasé about the whole thing that did I object to her stitching him up with just a local? This is how Adam ended up having half a bottle removed from his foot, and his heel being stitched back together with a darning needle, all while playing games on his phone and moaning that he'd been promised pizza but was now stuck in a boring hospital that didn't even have Wi-Fi. And all I could think was thank God for SPD.

On that positive note – and for once I'm being sincere because this was a genuine positive – here are a few suggestions if your child has any kind of sensory issues.

1. Relax

Remember, it's not your fault. I know I've said it before, but it's worth repeating. This isn't bad parenting, there isn't something going on at home (unless there is!), this is just how your child was made.

2. Accept you can't micro-manage your children

All you need to do is provide them with unconditional love, clothing, food and advice. Thereafter, it's their life and if they'd rather wear short sleeves than a coat and scarf in mid-winter, then that's their choice. You don't need to feel embarrassed or parent-shamed. You're doing a good job and giving your children everything they need.

3. Don't force your children to do anything they don't want to do

We have so many other areas of conflict in our home, we can live without another one, thank you very much. Give them choices and allow extra time for decisions to be made, but if they pick the one you think is wrong, go with it.

4. Be sympathetic

Keep in mind your child isn't doing this to annoy you. Well, I think mine are … but yours aren't. They don't want to be this way. And they really aren't lying or being difficult when they say their clothes are itchy or scratchy or twisty or tight(y). You wouldn't want to feel uncomfortable in your clothes, so why should they?

5. Note what they're wearing

If you take your child to the park, remember what colour their shoes are. If they mysteriously turn red, this isn't a miracle or a sign of the Second Coming. Call 999 immediately. Just whatever you do, don't buy red trainers!

12

E IS FOR EMBARRASSING PHOTOS

You've read about them, but now it's time to see them in Technicolor. I know at the very least you'll have been looking forward to seeing the photo of Zoe's shape test and Adam's magical T-shirt.

See you on the other side.

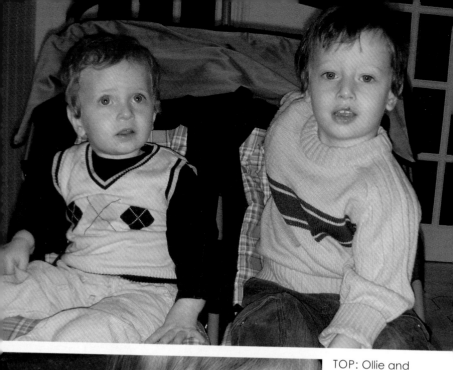

TOP: Ollie and Adam, aged two and three, in the double buggy we purchased after 'Butchergate'.

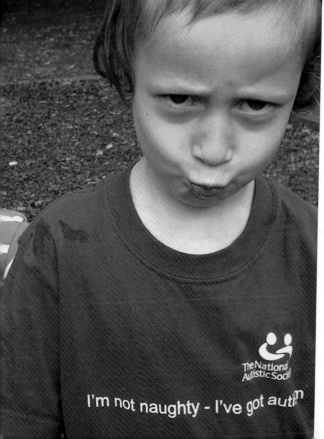

Adam in *the T-shirt*.

I'm not naughty - I've got autism

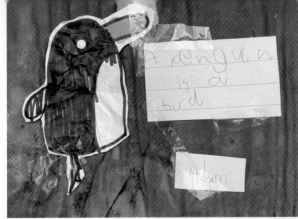

A penguin is a bird

Adam

When it comes to penguins, what more needs to be said?

Gemma with Zoe, the day she moved into our home in March 2011.

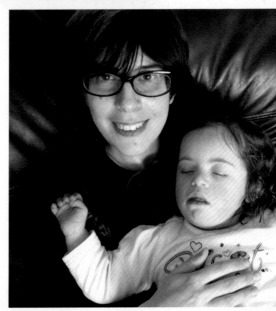

BELOW: Adam scaling Berkhamsted Castle like Spider-Man.

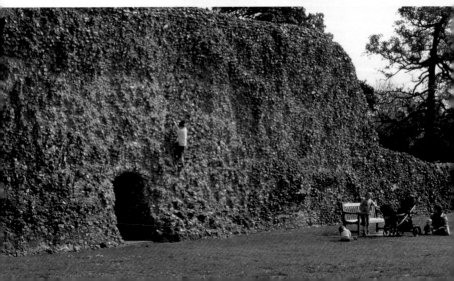

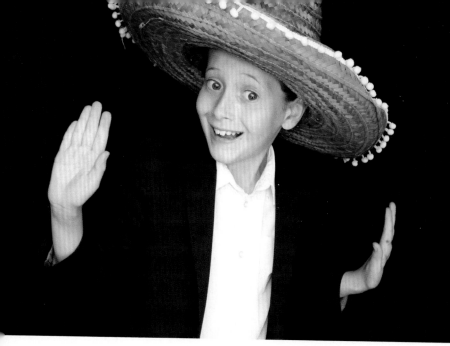

Dylan just being Dylan.

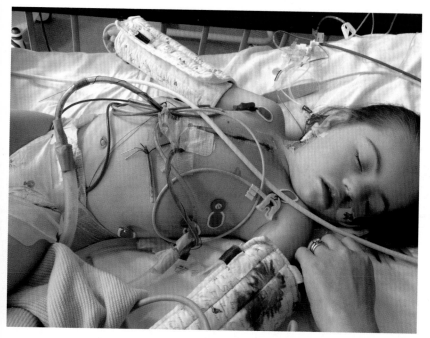

Seeing your child like this never gets easier. Zoe post
heart-op number two in July 2013.

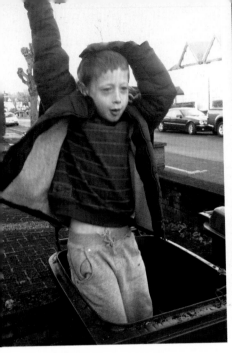

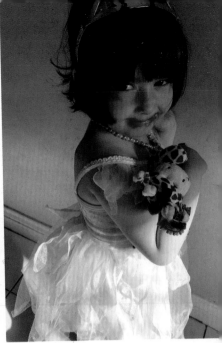

Adam playing in a wheelie bin.
Nothing odd about that.

The Bailey in all her glory. Here she
is aged four but going on 24.

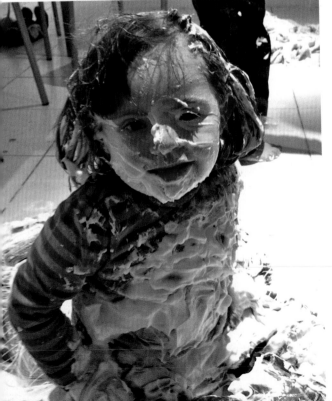

I made the mistake
of leaving a can of
shaving foam within
Zoe's reach. This
incident became
known as
'Foamgate'.

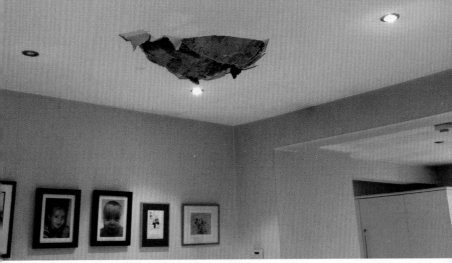

TOP: 'Please can everyone make sure they don't use our bathroom?' Famous last words before 'Toiletgate'.

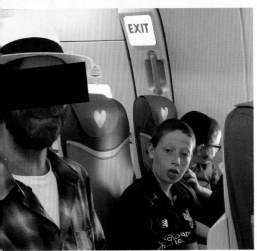

LEFT: Johnny Vine is all smiles at this point. Dylan is sitting on the other side of him about to unleash hell.

BELOW: Adam's *bar mitzvah* party. Some parents still refuse to talk to us following '*GTA*gate'.

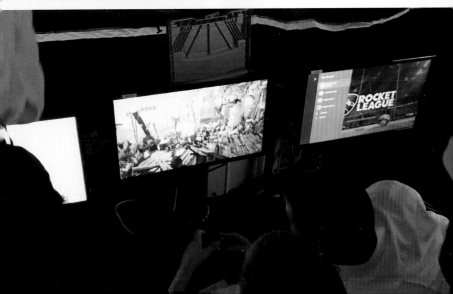

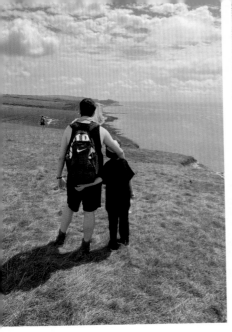

I love this photo so much.
Edward spending quality time
with his eldest brother, Adam.

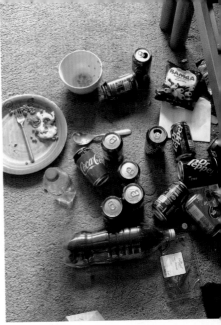

What I once pulled out from
under Adam's bed. Some of the
cans weren't even opened.

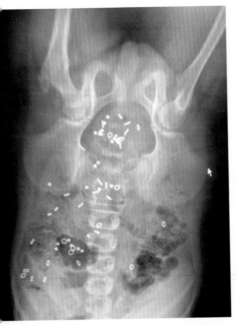

The X-ray that proves I correctly
administered Zoe's DIY shape-test.

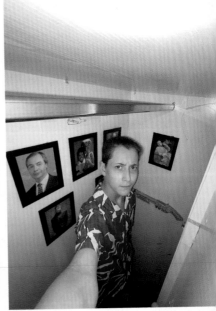

Dylan in The Nut Room. I don't
even know where to begin.

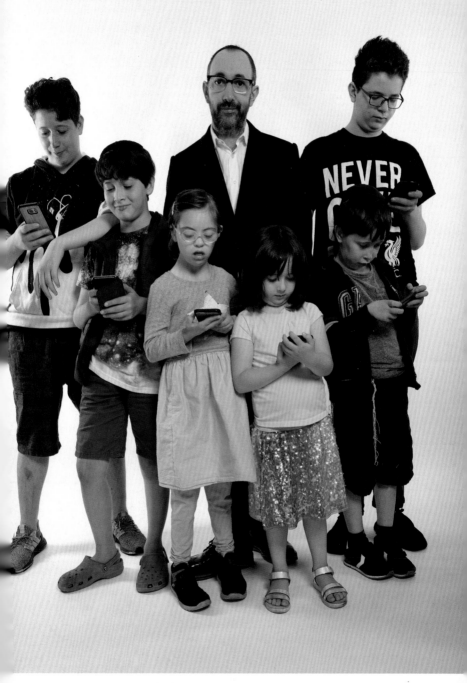

This photo sums up our house.
Broken charger cables not pictured.

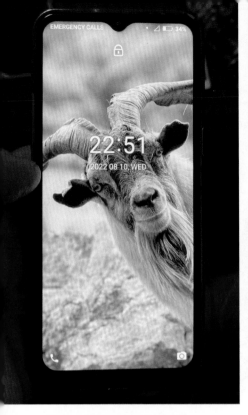

The wallpaper on Edward's phone. Brilliant.

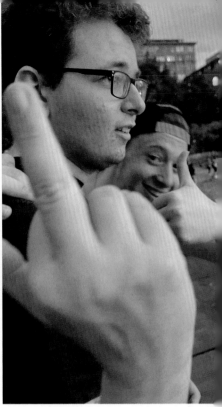

Teenage boys. Ollie and Adam in New York, summer 2022.

A rare photo looking like a regular family at Butlin's in April 2022.

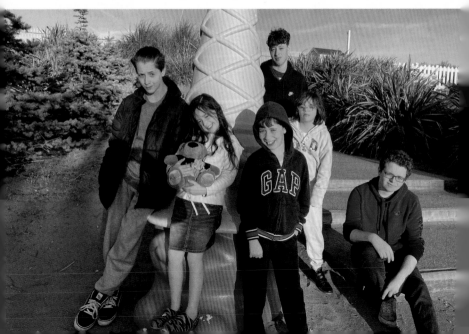

13

N IS FOR NO ROOM AT THE INN

For avoidance of doubt, this chapter is about our efforts trying to get our children, especially Adam, into school. It isn't about Jesus of Nazareth, although there are many signs he was neurodiverse. For a start, he apparently had an incredible knowledge of the Scriptures, and I imagine many annoying people would have approached Mary in the playground to ask if Jesus was a savant like that bloke in *Rain Man*. I just hope his parents – Mary, Joseph and possibly God; the jury's out – found Nazarene schools more accepting than we did, because nothing in my life has prompted me to ask 'Why hast thou forsaken me?' more than this tale of woe.

The sad reality is while schools have a duty to accept children with SEN and make reasonable adjustments on their behalf, many are resistant, to say the least. Even if they have a SENDCo and other professionals in place to help those with extra needs, some seem to view it as too much work and want to make sure there isn't a surfeit of *Zappas* in any one class. There are also financial considerations that come into play. In a September 2021 survey by the National Association of Head Teachers, 97 per cent of school leaders polled said that funding for SEND pupils was insufficient. Even if a child has an EHCP, it didn't seem to make much difference: 95 per cent claimed funding was still inadequate in these cases. The same poll revealed that over 80 per cent had been forced to pay for extra services, including speech and language therapy, educational psychologists and mental health support. Considering that in the not-too-distant past these services were provided by local councils, it's somewhat understandable that schools worry about the potential cost of *Zappas*. Of course, Jesus was lucky to live before austerity, and any cost of topping up his statement would have been offset by his ability to feed the multitude in the school lunchroom with just five loaves and two fish.

Whatever the reasons, the pain some parents feel on account of schools' unwillingness to accommodate their children is immeasurable. This is especially the case when you have a child like Adam, who hovers between two worlds. Football fans will know of those players like David Nugent and Robert Earnshaw who were too good for the Championship but not good enough for the Premier League. They could bang in over 20 goals a season in the second tier of English football, but would struggle to even reach double-figures playing against the likes of Liverpool, Manchester City and Chelsea in the top flight. This seems a very good metaphor for children such as Adam. He also fell between two tiers: mainstream and special schools. He didn't have sufficiently severe needs that would have merited him going to a special school like Zoe. However, neither was he someone like

Dylan, who could happily go to a regular school with a little additional support. Adam's EHCP acknowledged this fact. He was awarded 35 hours of LSA time – the same hours as Zoe – and it was evident from the description of his behaviour that he would be, in layman's terms, a bit of a handful.

Our attempts to get him into the school of our choice unfolded as follows:

May 2008

As he approached his fourth birthday, Adam was still at nursery and making slow but definite progress. His diagnosis was evident in the areas of social interaction, communication and speech, but his understanding was age-appropriate and he was completing work in line with his peers. We needed to decide where to send him next and hoped he could go to the same school where we intended to send Ollie, not least because it would make life a lot easier to have just one school run each morning. We aren't complete lunatics, although I accept much of what you've already read will suggest otherwise.

We'd briefly considered a specialist provision but the placement manager at the LEA (local education authority, in our case Barnet Council) in charge of Adam's statement had already decided this was not the way forward. The teachers from the council's early intervention service had been working with Adam for a year, so were able to make a decent assessment as to what setting would be most suitable. The upshot was the LEA decided we needed to name a mainstream school and unless we were minded to appeal to SENDIST (Special

Educational Needs and Disability Tribunal), this would be the end of the matter.

June 2008

No, this definitely wouldn't be the end of the matter. You see, when you name a school in your child's statement, they're then informed. And while it would be lovely to imagine they might think, 'Wonderful, we've been given the opportunity to welcome a child whose life we can impact for the better, and we're so looking forward to taking on the challenge,' this wasn't what happened in our case. Far from it, in fact.

Please bear in mind the following: all Adam's teachers and relevant professionals felt he could cope in a mainstream school. The LEA also informed us that the school had a past record of including children with ASD, and that BEAM were successfully working with other pupils.* Also remember, unless they can meet very stringent criteria, British schools are legally obliged to accept a child who has named them on their EHCP. Some will even consider it an honour to be entrusted with the care of a vulnerable child, although maybe that would have been asking a bit too much, especially considering this was Adam Blaker we were talking about.

It's common and good practice for schools to immediately get in touch with parents to discuss the transition, but we received no such contact. So we took the initiative

---

* Blimey, if I had a pound for every abbreviation in this book, well, it wouldn't be that much money, but it would at least pay for some more phone chargers.

and emailed them to request a meeting. No reply. Never ones to take a hint, we next phoned the school and asked to speak to the headteacher. We were told he was unavailable. Let's be honest, the warning signs were there.

Eventually, we received a phone call from the SENDCo, and thus started *Operation: Keep Adam Blaker Out of This School*. Their first step was to explain to us how the school was completely inappropriate for our son and to hope we'd change our minds. We said the LEA had highly recommended them, but she replied they must have confused the school with another. When we reminded the SENDCo that the specialist from BEAM visited the school every week, she promptly put the phone down while we were mid-sentence. It was already clear this wouldn't be a simple process.

The next stage of their plan was to completely fuck with our heads. They made an appointment for us to come in, but a few hours later called back to cancel it. I requested again to speak to the headteacher and was told once more that he was unavailable. When I asked if we could arrange a meeting, the administrator answered, 'I've been told to inform you there will be no meeting.' Nothing like being made to feel welcome.

Early July 2008

As my musical hero Morrissey once sang, 'The more you ignore me, the closer I get.'* So while many would have

---

* Musical hero, not political hero. Unfortunately, it feels necessary to give that caveat when it comes to Moz these days.

taken the hint, this only made us more determined. Moreover, due to Gemma's work, we knew our rights and understood that the actions of the school were legally discriminatory. Hence, we enlisted support from a parent advocate who specialised in ensuring children's entitlements are met and who on listening to our story so far was gobsmacked. She genuinely said this was one of the worst cases of discrimination she had ever heard, and we hadn't even set foot through the door of the school yet! We also consulted a lawyer who specialises in education and disability law, and who concurred that this was an open and shut case.

Sadly, no one had told the school, who now wrote to the LEA to make their case for refusing our son. Among the official reasons given was that Adam's attendance was not compatible 'with the efficient education of other children in the school'. Basically, this boy is going to disturb everyone so much that no one is going to be able to learn. The most chilling claim – outright gaslighting – was that they were 'perplexed as to why his parents feel that our busy mainstream classroom would be an appropriate placement' considering they had 'neither visited it nor discussed teaching methods' with the school. Yes, you really did read that correctly. We were being criticised for not having the meeting we had spent weeks begging for!

The school also cited health and safety concerns, maintaining that Adam's ASD would put other children at risk. Admittedly, some of this was based on lines in the EHCP that focused on his unruly or disruptive behaviour in the classroom. Yet they should have had enough professional experience of dealing with these documents to realise that the very nature of statements is to make the child appear as bad as possible, to ensure that it's granted in the first place. Besides, since the LEA was offering more than full-time LSA support, there was no reason why reasonable steps could not be taken by the school to prevent any incompatibility. The local authority was also offering extra help to ensure Adam's transition went smoothly, so it was no surprise when Barnet rejected their appeal. *Operation: Keep Adam Blaker Out of This School* had officially failed!!

Late July 2008

Not so fast. I sent an email to the headteacher asking if we could finally arrange a meeting, and received a startling reply. He said they would be appealing the LEA's decision to the secretary of state for education, and until the outcome of the appeal was known, they couldn't accede to our request to meet. Whether they thought they'd be successful or not is a moot point, but tellingly the email said the school would now be closing for the summer, and they didn't expect the DCSF (the Department of Children, Schools and Families, which has since been rebranded the Department of Education) to resolve the matter until mid-September or later.

At the very least, it didn't sound like Adam would be able to start school at the beginning of term. Evidently, their tactics now amounted to hoping that if heels were dragged sufficiently slowly then surely we'd give up and go elsewhere. Clearly, the school didn't know me and Gemma. We can be as stubborn as anyone, and there was no way we were giving up now. Not only that, but the LEA were also in touch with the DCSF to hurry them up and ensure Adam could attend school on the first day of term.

August 2008

For all our stubbornness and desire to be victorious, this was a truly horrible period. It had already taken so much out of us, both in terms of energy and time. All the emails and phone calls; the many discussions with Barnet, our advocate, and the lawyer. And now it was the summer holiday, and there was nothing we could do but hold tight and wait for a decision. We were also facing the real possibility that Adam would not have a school at the start of term. The LEA were very kind and offered home tuition from the BEAM teachers as a stopgap, and we tried as best we could to put this whole sorry situation to the back of our mind. But the pain didn't go away and there were constant reminders every time someone asked where Adam was going in September.

During this time, we also saw the documents the school submitted to the DCSF which included the most extraordinary claim yet. Are you sitting down? No, really, I feel you need to be prepared for this one. The school claimed – I shit you not!! – that since they knew I worked in television, they were concerned we were only pushing for Adam's entry so he could be sent in wearing covert cameras to gather footage for a TV documentary about the treatment of SEN children in the classroom. I really do hope you were sitting down!

Just to be clear, I'm not making this up. They thought my little Adam – a four-year-old boy with ASD – was the next Roger Cook or Donal MacIntyre. What this claim was based on, I have no idea. It's true I did work in TV, but I wrote and produced comedy. Writing occasional knob gags for Graham Norton to say on Channel 4 hardly counts as investigative journalism, so I don't know how this would have entered their heads. If ever there was a sign of what we were dealing with, this was it.

8 September 2008

As we were warned would happen, the term began and there was still no decision. It was a sad day seeing other children heading off to start their school years. We did our best to bury our heads in the sand, and avoided photos of kids looking all cute and excited doing what Adam should have been doing too. We already felt his behaviour was deteriorating and we worried about him going backwards after the amazing progress of the past six months. This seemed a real danger if he were to continue missing an important part of his education. Neither did we want to mope around the house, so we took our boys to LEGOLAND for the day and tried to have a fun day out. And it was there, while queuing for one of the rides, that we got the call we'd been waiting for. The secretary of state for children, schools and families had decreed that the school would have to take Adam.

This was such a moment of joy and relief, and looking back I still can't believe it was Ed Balls MP who ultimately made this decision about our son. This is the man who on 28 April 2011 would prompt an annual event known as Ed Balls Day when he accidentally tweeted the words 'Ed Balls'. In 2016, he became a laughing stock again when he danced to 'Gangnam Style' on *Strictly Come Dancing*, a performance the *Guardian* claimed 'we can never unsee'. But for me, Ed Balls will always be a hero. He's the man who finally told this school to shut the fuck up and take our son, and for that, he will forever have our gratitude.

9 September 2008

I wish I could say this was the end of 'Admissionsgate', but I'm sure you'll have guessed this wasn't the case. After previously refusing to meet with me and Gemma, the school now wanted an urgent meeting to see if they could persuade us that this was the wrong place for Adam. They also said they couldn't accept him until a suitable LSA was found; this would need to be advertised, and there was no guarantee the right person would apply. They even threated seeking a judicial review of the decision through the High Courts or going to the House of Lords.

The DCSF were not amused with this response and threatened sanctions if a start date wasn't given immediately. The LEA even raised the salary of the proposed LSA significantly, to ensure the best person would be found. And so, on Monday 22 September 2008 Adam finally started at the school of our choice.

The obvious question is why on earth did we persist with our attempts to send Adam to this school. They'd made it abundantly clear that they didn't want him and were willing to do almost anything to stop him attending. Some people love it when the object of their desire plays hard to get, but this was outright hostility. Many friends doubted our sanity and wondered why we didn't just go elsewhere. Surely, as some pointed out, even if we were to be successful in the battle, we would ultimately lose the war, because the school would be so resentful towards us that Adam wouldn't receive the kindness and patience that he required to thrive.

It's a fair question and one that we asked ourselves at the time. We're both incredibly stubborn people. I've joked that if I told Gemma her hair was on fire, she'd rather burn than heed any point of mine regarding her appearance. So we did discuss this to ensure we weren't digging our heels in to make a point, especially considering it would be at the expense of our son's education. And with my hand on my heart, I can tell you we were one hundred per cent convinced this was the right setting for Adam. We had thoroughly researched it and spoken to parents of other children at the school, including several with SEN. We had previously visited when it came to choosing a school for Ollie. It was an excellent primary school, with good reports from OFSTED, and everything we'd seen had made us think these plaudits were well deserved. We also felt we knew our son better than anyone and genuinely believed that his needs were not incompatible with mainstream school. On the contrary, we thought – no, we knew – that with the right support he'd flourish in this environment.

What's more, I hate to be the guy that says, 'I told you so,' but we were proved right in the end. And a huge part of the credit for that needs to be given to the school. After this horrible battle, and with our relationship with them at an all-time low, the headteacher called us into his office and said he wanted to start again. Thereafter, he was never anything less than charming and helpful, as were the SENDCo, Adam's teachers and his staggeringly patient LSAs. For our part we did everything to show we were grateful and that we were realistic about what Adam could achieve. We didn't expect miracles and were willing to put our trust in them to do what they felt was best. After all, we'd fought this battle because we believed they were an exceptional school, so it would have been nonsensical to then micro-manage or second-guess every decision they made. We listened and followed their advice, and they could see we were hands-on parents who wanted the best for our son. We also knew we needed to get over our hurt because otherwise it wouldn't have worked. And so, remarkably, we built bridges with the school, Adam was there for seven mostly happy years, and he left with many friends and good memories. Plus, I won a BAFTA for that covert documentary that Adam helped me make about London's primary schools. Well, that part isn't true, but the rest is.

It would be great to argue that this was a unique situation, but I think it's much more common than you'd imagine. And it's not just schools, as local authorities themselves seem to wage war on the parents of SEN children. Only recently I read an article on the ITV News website that claimed councils are spending hundreds of thousands of pounds fighting legal battles with families, only to lose almost every time. For example, in the last four years, councils in the East of England have had more than a thousand appeals lodged by parents unhappy with their child's EHCP, and of those, the authorities won just 51, equivalent to losing 95 per cent of cases. That's a win ratio that makes Frank Lampard's stint at Everton look successful.

This chapter has been the hardest for me to write so far. I've gone back through documents and emails that I haven't looked at in years and have reminded myself of some extremely miserable moments. I hope I've made it sufficiently amusing to avoid this becoming the mis-lit I promised not to write. At the very least, the story about the covert filming should have made you chuckle, because it certainly did me. But as with the rest of this book, I want to be positive, and I share this traumatic tale to help rather than to frighten you. So, let's end with some suggestions if any of this happens to you.

1. Keep calm

Easier said than done, but schools and LEAs will rely on you losing your patience and giving up.

2. Check your motivation

Make sure you're certain you want to fight and that you're doing it for the right reasons. It's tempting to be stubborn for the sake of it. Only continue if you believe this is the right course of action for your child.

3. Know your rights

Disability legislation is on your side and on the side of your child. Be sure you're aware of what you're entitled to and what you should expect when it comes to schools.

4. If it all gets too much, find a parent advocate

Parent advocates are usually free of charge and are the Hannibal Smith and B. A. Baracus of the SEN world. They're able to come and resolve the problems you can't; and pity the fool at any school who messes with them. Thankfully they're easier to find than the A-Team, not basing themselves in the Los Angeles underground – unless they are parent advocates in Los Angeles, in which case they may do – and you won't need to drug anyone's milk.

5. If the shit hits the fan, seek legal support

There are many specialists in education and disability law, and they may well be happy to work *pro bono*.* Ask your parent advocate to put you in touch with an appropriate lawyer.

---

* That means free. It's nothing to do with U2.

6. Try to build bridges

If you go through a situation like ours, do your utmost to mend fences with your child's school.* Be realistic about what they can do: they're not miracle workers! Gifts and notes of appreciation will go a long way to helping too. And if you find yourself constantly second-guessing and micro-managing them, then that's probably a red flag that this is the wrong school after all.

7. Don't hang on to the hurt

We had such a harrowing journey, but it was vital to try to forget about it and move on. And I did, at least until HarperCollins asked me to write about it, which has brought all the pain back. Cheers for that!

Good luck. And if all else fails, you could always send your child to school wearing covert cameras and film what's going on. Either that, or move to Nazareth and see if their schools are as welcoming as I think they were a couple of thousand years ago.

---

* I know I just suggested building bridges, but I think mending fences is better. Fences tend to be much smaller than bridges, and by and large, mending something is less work than building it from scratch. I bet if you asked Isambard Kingdom Brunel, he'd say he regrets not getting into fence repair and having more leisure time.

14

J IS FOR JUST NOT MADE FOR SCHOOL

After all the hassles of getting a child into school, it would be lovely to think you could now put your feet up and enjoy the fruits of your labour. We've already covered the problem of relentless meetings, but there's an even bigger issue, and it's a truth that in some ways feels unsayable. Put simply, some children just aren't made for school. There, I said it.

This goes especially for those with additional needs. For many it's too rigid, too challenging, too noisy. If Dylan finds the sound of Coco Pops too loud, what chance does he have coping with a hectic classroom or playground?! It's true that schools are required to make reasonable adjustments for children with SEN and, of course, many will. Your child may also be entitled to one-on-one LSA time. We've been very fortunate in that regard, and I don't want to appear ungrateful. But even with all the extra help in the world, it could be that your *Zappa* is never going to find that school is for them. Perhaps we need to accept that education only works for those who are good at education, and in the case of many children, that fundamentally isn't them.

Adam, for example, couldn't quite settle after primary school, moving several times during his secondary years. He's now been inside more schools than an OFSTED inspector. It was only when he went to college for a Level 1 course in Introduction to Social Services, and to do his GCSE retakes – and then retake the retakes – that he really started to thrive. He completed the course and moved onto a Level 2 programme in Sports, which was no small achievement and one of which we were immensely proud. But while I'd love to argue that his previous schools were at fault, I'm not sure any secondary school would have been right for Adam. He thrived eventually, but only in the very different atmosphere of college, and only after his 16th birthday, by which point he had matured immensely.

Now in his later teens, Adam has finally grasped that he must take some responsibility for his own education. Previously, he took a completely passive role. I recall Gemma receiving a text from Adam, one lunchtime. It was a photo of his Science test and it had a large 0 per cent written in red pen at the top. The picture was accompanied by the following message from Adam to Gemma:

Y didnt u revyse! This is yr folt idiot 💀💀💀💀💀💀

It says a lot that our first instinct was to email Adam's Science teacher with an apology for not revising.

On visits to his primary school for parents' evening, each class would have their work put on display. We quickly learnt that to find Adam's contribution, we'd need to walk to the very back of the classroom, where his efforts would be hidden from other mums and dads, lest they think this is the level of learning and write letters of complaint. One highlight was a project the class had completed about birds of the world. The walls were covered with impressive artwork featuring lavish detail about the feeding habits, average weights and wing spans of parrots, owls, eagles and so on. Last of all was a surprisingly decent drawing of a penguin, no doubt mostly the work of Adam's LSA. Alongside it had been glued a small scrap of paper with a few words written in pencil. These were just about legible and simply read: 'A penguin is a bird.' Who needs statistics and details? A penguin is a bird and that's all you need to know. We instantly fell in love with this piece and still have it safely stored for posterity at home.*

Dylan has also matured and found his feet at secondary school, but seeing that he inhabits the bizarre world of his own brain, things haven't always been simple. A few years ago I took him to see his future school, and on arrival we were each handed a sticky label on which to write our names. And for reasons best known to himself, whereas I wrote Ashley Blaker, Dylan wrote in big felt tip, 'Bruce Wayne'. I was baffled.

'Dylan, why have you written Bruce Wayne?! That's not your name!'

He looked at me and with an entirely straight face replied, 'How do you know?'

'How do I know?! Because I've lived with you for the past ten years, and I was at your birth, and I'm sure I'd

---

* And if you haven't seen it already, turn back to the photos and marvel at its uncomplicated genius.

remember if when the midwife asked, "What's his name?" instead of saying Dylan Blaker I'd said, "Bruce Wayne".'

This stopped Dylan in his tracks. He paused momentarily before saying, 'Well, don't tell anyone.' I guess it turns out Batman was in Edgware after all.

I'm not sure which visit to secondary school was worse: Dylan's, with his non-stop surrealism, or Adam's, which was characterised by an almost total lack of communication. When the headteacher took us around one of Adam's many schools a few years earlier – they all blur into one after a while – Adam said almost nothing until the very end, when the head asked what he thought of it. To which he simply replied, 'Dunno.' And if you're not the parent of a monosyllabic *Zappa*, that translates as, 'This school is very impressive, I think the standards of both teaching and facilities are outstanding, and I'd be only too happy to attend.'

Even now, Dylan has some way to go before he reaches Adam's level of maturity – talk about a low bar! – and understanding that he needs to take responsibility for his schoolwork. Last term, there was a major panic before he left for the bus one morning. Dylan was yelling, 'Where's my History project?'

I pointed out this was quite a misleading question because it would imply he'd done it in the first place.

'Why didn't you remind me?' he screamed in reply. I flashed back to the previous evening when Gemma had punctuated every ten minutes by saying, 'Have you done your homework yet?' Dylan meanwhile spent the entire night filling latex gloves with water and bursting them into the bathtub. Unless his project was on the history of immaturity and time-wasting in post-Brexit Britain, it would appear his mother's words went unheeded.

Some *Zappas*, like Zoe, attend special schools, and this is a whole different ball game because the environment is designed just for them. That's not to say these children will be immune from any issues, but I can only write about our experiences, and by and large Zoe has always gone to school very cheerfully. She loves everything about it, from the teachers to her classmates, and while over the years I've found fault with various things, Zoe has been consistently happy – and that's the main thing. Consequently, I've not bothered to raise most of my concerns with the school. I also don't want to be called in for a *Discussion about Mr Blaker's opinions with a view to him becoming a more grateful parent transition meeting*.

However, our experiences with Zoe are totally unlike those with our boys, who have only attended mainstream schools. And for most parents of *Zappas*, this is the challenge. For one thing, being the parents of children with SEN puts you in a particularly vulnerable space when it comes to taking offence. We realised early on with our autistic boys that if we were ever going to have any friends in the playground, we had to stop using every conversation as a reason to get upset. We'd listen as other parents bemoaned the fact their kid hadn't finished the last book of Harry Potter, knowing full well our boys were still on phonics. Other mums and dads proudly received their children's artistic efforts, and all ours were done by teaching assistants. Very nicely, I might add, as that beautiful penguin should prove. We needed to overcome all that, and at least be grateful that only making Pot Noodles every night meant we had very little washing-up.

We also need to constantly encourage our darling children to go to schools that are designed solely for *Coldplays*. I'm almost totally skint from buying rewards for our boys. I've even bought presents for a child because he got five per cent on a maths test. Obviously, it's a terrible mark by any normal standards, but it was a huge improvement on the previous term's score of two per cent, so deserved to be recognised.

The schools also use rewards to try to elicit good behaviour and better learning. So on top of the non-stop meetings, we've found ourselves being dragged back to school for assemblies to see one of our sons receive an award they've clearly made up to encourage him. I know they mean well, but it's also slightly humiliating. Gemma and I would sit alongside the parents of other children who were receiving prizes. They would all look so proud, as well they might, but the two of us looked rather more sheepish. We'd been here before, so knew what was coming. One boy would be called up to the front to be given a prize for breaking the school's 100m record. Everyone would clap. Then a second child would be invited to the stage for raising over £2,000 for Cancer Research. Very deserving, and again, everyone applauds. Then the headteacher would clear his throat. 'And finally, a prize goes to Dylan Blaker for remembering his own name.' Which he probably didn't anyway, because he thinks his name is Bruce Wayne.

I've no doubt the schools have the best of intentions here. Again, I don't want to come across as ungrateful to people who are making some effort to differentiate. But it's rather chastening to watch the other parents give us weak smiles, as they half-heartedly applaud our son's meagre achievements. And this isn't only about me and my damaged pride, as important as that may be! More significant is the question of what lesson these unearned rewards teach our children. Probably that you don't need to try too hard, because so long as you turn up, the teachers will say, 'Brilliant effort,' give you a prize and allow you to eat some unhealthy snacks. I'd love this book to win a real award for being good, but if it's rubbish, the head of HarperCollins won't create one and then buy me a packet of crisps.*

Naturally, these prizes for almost nothing are even more problematic when there are five other children in the house, because now everyone else wants a reward as well. A few years ago, after Dylan managed some huge achievement like putting his gloves on the correct hands, I bought him a set of Transformer toys, which led to a traumatic episode known in our house as 'Transformergate'. I really don't want to revisit it, but let's just say everyone wanted some of these toys. Then, after Dylan counted them and realised one of his Transformers was missing, it led to an even uglier mess than the *Transformers* movies. Shrewdly, we didn't tell his teachers that it turns out Dylan can count, because that would have meant attending yet another school assembly. Of course, barely two weeks after 'Transformergate', I discovered three 'robots in disguise' now disguised down the back of the sofa, as everyone had moved on to fighting over something else.

Even when we aren't going in for a meeting or to see our sons receive a newly invented prize, it's rare for a day

---

* If you're reading this, Mr Collins, I'm fond of McCoy's Salt & Malt Vinegar. Just saying.

to go by without a phone call from one of their teachers about some kind of 'incident'. I've been tempted to send our boys to school wearing a sign around their neck saying, 'Please do NOT call my parents. This really is just the way I am. Do not be alarmed. And DON'T call home. They're working/sleeping/busy with a huge argument over who should be taking the calls from school!' The only reason I haven't is because I know it wouldn't work. As noted earlier, there's nothing teachers love more than a paper trail; not even summer holidays or Christmas presents from parents. So if there's an 'incident' you can expect a call, regardless of whether you begged them not to.

When there are multiple *Zappas* in a class, 'incidents' are common. Adam had four others in his class: one with a diagnosis and an EHCP, and three more whose parents refused to believe they were anything other than *Coldplays*. I knew better, simply because these kids were friends with Adam. Who needs to spend years at university, training to be a child psychiatrist?! If a boy is friends with Adam, I can guarantee you he has ASD or ADHD, or most likely both.

Probably the most serious of these classroom occurrences led to the swift formation of a WhatsApp group for the mothers of all five boys, even the three mums with their heads in the sand. Suitably, the group was named 'The Incident', and I still thank God that for some reason the dads weren't invited to join. After reading the progressively more hysterical messages, we went to ask Adam what exactly had happened. We found him in his room under a pile of old copies of the *Beano*, and he delivered his version of events while keeping his eyes permanently fixed on the screen of his Nintendo DS.*

'One-Word Freedman stole my crisps. Then Monotone Williams said he had to give them back, but One-Word Freedman said no way. Then Only-Eats-Rice-Cakes Davis stuck a pen down Monotone Williams's ear and One-Word Freedman joined in. Then Faraway-Look Daniels said our cat was stupid. Then Monotone Williams said at least the cat was cleverer than Faraway-Look Daniels. Then One-Word Freedman said you weren't funny, which I didn't really care about but also, I do really care.'

I'd turn this into a comic character, but I fear Vicky Pollard got there first. Suffice to say, after visiting Adam's bedroom we were none the wiser about what had tran-spired. Gemma related this to the WhatsApp group, while I sat quietly, trying to get over the fact that Adam's friend One-Word thinks I'm not funny. Even if it's from a nine-year-old *Zappa*, us comedians never like a bad review.

Regrettably, once your child gets a reputation for being involved in 'incidents', you will receive more phone calls about their alleged involvement in 'incidents'. I'm by no means suggesting my children are always blame-less, but there have been several cases of mistaken identity. Eight years ago, Adam's teacher rang to fill me in on something that had happened in the playground. It was the usual charge sheet: destruction of property, wilful disregard of school rules, blatant rudeness (to both a teacher and another pupil) and general vandalism. I

---

* NB names have been changed to protect the less than innocent.

pointed out that for some reason violent intimidation was missing, and we agreed that a lack of violence did suggest Adam hadn't been involved. The teacher promptly apologised and hung up, though not before I took the opportunity to suggest One-Word Freedman was the real culprit. That'll teach him for claiming I wasn't funny, the little shit!

The most remarkable of all the phone calls from school has gone down in Blaker family mythology and is known as 'Escortgate'. This was the occasion when Adam's teacher told us they were very concerned about him because during a creative writing lesson he had written that he wanted to hire an escort. There's so much that's bizarre about this story that to this day I'm puzzled why the school thought it necessary to mention it.

- Our son was eight years old.
- He had no knowledge of the sex industry.
- He was receiving £2 a week pocket money, which I imagine wouldn't go very far when it comes to the oldest profession.*

Typically, the first thing the school did was ask if anything was going on at home. Maybe they imagined my evenings involved inviting round sex workers, and now our son wanted a piece of the action. Then, Gemma and I were invited into school for a *Transition to banning the discussion of call girls planning meeting*. And yes, there

---

* I've never had cause to find out and I don't want to google 'How much would an escort cost?' in case anyone checks my internet search history.

was a box of tissues on the table, appropriate on several counts.

When they showed us what they laughably called his 'piece of work', there was a line that admittedly, if you squinted and looked at it for long enough, like one of those old Magic Eye posters, could possibly – and even then, only possibly – have read 'hire an escort'. However, it could just as easily have been 'find an escargot', and Adam was hinting at a love of edible snails. Then again, it might have read 'love MC Escher', suggesting that this eight-year-old wanted to share his fondness for visual illusions and paradoxical perspectives. Frankly, it could have been almost anything, including, 'I want to hire an Escort, because it's a decent family motor, economical on fuel, and even 20 years old would still be better than the piece of junk my father drives.'

Worst of all, no one had thought to ask Adam what he had written and had preferred jumping to conclusions. When we finally enquired, he replied, 'We had to write words, but I couldn't think of any words, so I just wrote some letters because letters make up words.' Which is the most brilliantly autistic approach to schoolwork I've ever heard. And so just as an infinite number of monkeys could knock out the complete works of Shakespeare, give Adam Blaker a pencil and tell him to write some random letters, and you might get something that looks like a request for a lady of the night. At least in the end we got an apology, and so, appropriately enough, the story of Adam and the escort did conclude with a happy ending.

Small mercies, perhaps, but for all Adam's bad behaviour and lack of interest in education, he never refused to attend school. I know of several *Zappas* who have hated it to such an extent that they would do anything to get out of going. Tragically, one boy was so unhappy, he cut the buttons off his school shirts in the hope this would mean he'd have to stay at home. I'm very grateful we've never had a child suffering in that way. The nearest we got was Dylan, who would much rather stay home and read comics, but usually isn't sufficiently imaginative to come up with anything better than, 'I don't feel well, can I have the day off?' The best he could do was the following claim, made one morning, five minutes before it was time for him to head off to school:

> I watched a video on YouTube that said they did an experiment in the United States where some children went to school and some stayed at home just watching TV, and apparently the ones that stayed at home watching TV ended up knowing more than the ones that went to school because you can actually learn a lot from watching quiz shows like *Jeopardy*, and they'll probably get better jobs in the future because knowing things impresses the kind of people who give you jobs whereas exams don't really mean very much because most jobs don't actually involve things like Geography and Chemistry.

I pointed out that this reputed experiment was in the US while we live in the UK, so tough luck, you're going to school, and that was pretty much that. I'd previously tried to argue that doing things we hate is good preparation for the responsibilities of real life. I then realised I was painting such a miserable vision of adulthood that it was best to insist he went to school without trying to make any case for its benefits.

But to get back to the title of this chapter, I've now concluded after many years of pain that perhaps some children just aren't made for school, and rather than let that upset me, it has allowed me to go easy on myself and the children. Not to give up – well, not totally, anyway – but to accept that formal education isn't for everyone. When he was in primary school, Adam's LSA would often call, saying things like, 'I'm worried about Adam.' In terms of frequency, this line was beaten only by, 'Mr Blaker, there's been an "incident".' And what usually worried her was that Adam didn't seem capable of following through on anything. That he'd start his work with the best of intentions, but then his energy would tail off and he'd find himself distracted by something else. He'd then want food and would come up with any excuse not to complete the original task. Yet while I don't want to minimise Adam's struggles and the diagnosis that underpins them, isn't that most of us? I've started writing numerous books over the years, and it's a near miracle that you're now holding in your hand the first one I've completed.

Adam knew what was expected of him. If I ever asked him what he was going to do at school today he'd roll his eyes and with total boredom chant his answer: 'Try-my-best-school-is-important-put-in-the-effort-that's-all-that-matters-be-polite-to-adults-stop-spending-my-lunch-money-on-gum-stop-taking-fake-weapons-into-school-keep-my-clothes-on-at-all-times.'

Regardless of his additional needs, why should we expect any more from children than we do from ourselves? We all have days when we can't be bothered, lose focus and don't complete our jobs. We have hundreds of unanswered emails; we ignore the cleaning; we don't stick with our plan to go to the gym; and we can't delay gratification, so polish off a packet of Milky Way Magic Stars in the middle of the afternoon. Yet while we allow ourselves days when it doesn't happen, we don't extend this compassion to our kids. We expect them to give their best and be focused all the time, then get frustrated when they act just like us.

Given my children's capacity to avoid working when expected to, it's not surprising every parent's evening I've ever attended has involved teachers saying lines like:

> The thing with Edward is he's like all the Blaker
> children I've taught. He's a lovely boy, well behaved
> [we both know they're stretching the truth here,
> but they tend to take pity on us], enthusiastic and
> curious. There's just one thing: he seems to feel
> that the normal rules don't apply to him.

I've heard all kinds of stories over the years. If the teacher sets six questions, our sons will do seven. If the teacher asks the class to write a diary, our boys produce a newspaper article. If the teacher wants the class to say the Jewish morning prayers, our boys have their shoes off and are bowing to Mecca. Is this the *Zappa* in them or just good old Blaker belligerence? The more I think about it, the more I'm convinced they're the same thing.

Is following your own rules so bad anyway? We often praise real innovators and avant-garde creatives for ignoring convention and marching to the beat of their own drum. Maybe, rather than despairing, we should be proud that we're raising such non-conformists. A refusal to follow the rules could hold one back in many aspects of adult life, but it hasn't prevented some people reaching the top of their profession. Many articles I've read about Boris Johnson have noted that everyone, from his masters at Eton and beyond, said the same of the former PM: that he felt the normal rules didn't apply to him. Clearly, Boris isn't the best role model, and I must stress my children display this trait in a more charming and less calculating fashion. 'Partygate' was a blatant breach of Boris's own rules and a fuck-you to the country; 'Papier-mâchégate' was only a fuck-you to Dylan's teachers, and even then, we've never truly got to the bottom of it, so I don't feel I should comment any further. My point is that if Boris Johnson can somehow get to 10 Downing Street despite thinking the normal rules don't apply, perhaps there's still hope for the Blakers. Adam has already been Leader of the Opposition to most of his teachers and, come to think of it, both his parents, so perhaps he could yet surprise us all and become leader of the nation.

And on that optimistic and slightly frightening note, here are some final thoughts to remember when it comes to *Zappas* and mainstream schools.

1. Relax

I think I've said this at the end of nearly every chapter, but is there a more important suggestion in this book? Be kind to yourself. If you can't get your child motivated for school, it isn't your fault. Unless it is, but it probably isn't.

2. School isn't for everyone

It works for most, but there are enough people without additional needs who have left early and been perfectly successful. Richard Branson, Seth Rogan, Steve Jobs, Quentin Tarantino, Alan Sugar and many others have done OK for themselves, so your child can too. Perhaps one day we'll see Adam on TV, telling a room full of wannabe apprentices that he doesn't like liars, cheats or bullshitters, though judging by his friends, he does.

3. Make sure your child's school differentiates for them

They have a duty to make reasonable adjustments for children with SEN, and if for some reason – laziness, ineptitude, stubbornness – they're not as accommodating as they should be, don't be shy about requesting a meeting. You could really turn the tables and even bring your own tissues.

4. Don't fall out with your child's school

For sure, you should push them to make reasonable adjustments, but do your best to keep them onside and to build a solid working relationship. This won't be easy if you've had a fight to get your child accepted, but even after all our issues, we formed very strong ties with the teachers and LSAs who worked with Adam in primary school. Our group emails became a kind of support group for fellow sufferers of our eldest son's behaviour.

5. Don't compare your child to their peers

A sure-fire way to make yourself unhappy is to pay attention to how many *Peter and Jane* books everyone else's child has read. When it comes to the playground, it's best to have selective hearing, so invest in some AirPods and whack the music up as high as it goes. You won't be able to hear the other mums and dads, and if you play the music at full volume, you'll damage your hearing sufficiently that you won't be able to hear them even when you don't have any music on.

6. Don't be too quick to blame schools

Adam moved several times, and it was only on reaching college that he began to thrive. Was his later success a sign that his previous schools were shit? In some cases, it was. But more importantly, he needed time to mature, and it was only in his later teens that things began to fall into place. So stay calm; there's plenty of time to go, and the future may well be rosier.

15

T IS FOR TRIPS AND VACATIONS

Cliff Richard famously sang about a summer holiday being all fun and laughter, with no worries and dreams coming true. Well, yes, I'm sure a holiday is fun when you're a 'Bachelor Boy'. Unfortunately, my experiences have been very different to Sir Cliff's, and I've realised that it doesn't matter whether the sun shines brightly, because taking my lot on vacation is such hard work that I've sometimes regretted it before we've even reached the airport.

First, let's get one thing straight. Something that feels slightly taboo to say but that I'm convinced everyone secretly agrees with. And this is that holidays with children – *Zappas* or *Coldplays* – aren't enjoyable. If you're a parent, a holiday would be to go away *without* your kids. Have some adult time and recharge your batteries before getting back to the grind. Some people are fortunate enough to do this, perhaps with the help of grandparents. But going away *with* your children? Why would anyone subject themselves to that?! It's just all the normal hassles of parenting but somewhere else.

Actually, it's even harder since you've got none of the creature comforts of home, and are in a location where it's not as easy to monitor little ones and keep them safe.

I'm convinced people only persist in taking their kids away because either a. they feel under pressure to do so having seen photos of smug bastards 'enjoying' their holidays on social media or b. they *are* the smug bastards who post photos of their family holidays on social media to make the rest of us feel like shit.

Now that's out the way, let's talk about holidays with *Zappas*, because if going away with *Coldplays* is no fun, then this is fun minus 500.* Most of our family vacations have been in the UK and not even involved any of the enormous hassles of air travel, yet they've still proved hugely challenging.

Our first was in April 2008 when we took our then three boys – Adam (3), Ollie (2), and Dylan (six months) – to a holiday camp in Leicestershire. Certainly not Sir Cliff's idea of a summer holiday destination, seeing that we'd chosen a location as far away from the sea as almost anywhere in the UK. Plus, being April, it was more of an Easter holiday and I imagine this devout Christian wouldn't have been impressed that we spent Good Friday not at church but in a drizzly park in Ashby-de-la-Zouch frightening the locals.

My first inkling that this was a mistake was when I tried to load up the car. The double buggy we'd purchased to ensure Adam didn't run off was still very much required, but considering we had a six-month-old in his own pushchair, it was either leave it or buy another car.

---

* As measured on the official Blaker Fun-o-meter.

We were going to have to go old school and keep our wits about us if we wanted to avoid a repeat of 'Butchergate'. To keep Adam happy, we also needed to bring as many of his favourite things as possible, including a carload of *Thomas* trains for him to line up. Half the residents of Sodor seemed to be gathered in my boot, along with four separate playsets and three carrycases – one for Ollie and the other two for Adam to hold in each of his hands – leaving almost no room for me to pack any clothes.

No offence to residents of the East Midlands, but let's be honest and admit Leicestershire in April isn't exactly the Caribbean or Dubai. Yet I can't truthfully say it would have been easier anywhere else in the world. Perhaps the sight of wildebeest grazing on the Serengeti or the sun setting on the New York skyline would have made it visually more appealing, but the fundamental issues would have remained. We were parenting our difficult autistic child away from the home in which he was happy – well, as happy as he could be, given his frustrations around communication – and in which it was more feasible to prevent him endangering himself and/or others. This was less than a year after the disappearance of Madeleine McCann, and every parent in the country was now obsessively watching their children on vacation. We shared that communal paranoia, but with the added complication of trying to monitor a very energetic boy with ASD and no interest in staying where we wanted him to, all without his buggy because it wouldn't fit in the car.

It was a sufficiently arduous week that we didn't attempt it again for another seven years. It was still an Easter rather than summer holiday – sorry, Sir Cliff – but at least we'd learnt our lesson and decided to opt for a more exotic locale than Leicestershire. This time we were just outside Milton Keynes. I bet you were expecting me to say the Bahamas.* We at least upgraded our accommodation from a holiday camp to a hotel. It might not have been the Ritz, but it was a Grade II-listed manor house that was apparently the birthplace of the former *Blue Peter* gardening expert Percy Thrower. Quite why he was born there rather than in hospital is unclear, but my guess is the Throwers were also given the wrong phone number to call.

For all the positive differences, other changes to our lives made this holiday even harder. By April 2014 Adam was easier, having matured a little and crucially having been prescribed drugs. However, Dylan had now been diagnosed with ASD, and we were joined this time by a five-year-old Zoe, a three-year-old Edward and an eight-week-old Bailey. By this point we had an eight-seater Toyota Previa to accommodate all the children, but still needed a second car to fit all the teddies, blankets, buggies, toys, books, and so many arts and craft materials that had Percy Thrower still resided there he'd have thought he was back on *Blue Peter*.

I don't want to be overly negative about this holiday. The hotel was near all the leisure facilities in Milton Keynes, and it was great to be able to give some freedom to the children by letting Adam, Ollie and Dylan wander off to explore the plentiful grounds. The post-Maddy

---

* That would have been a particularly depressing metaphor for Emily Perl Kingsley: we were expecting a week in the Caribbean and ended up in Buckinghamshire.

terror had eased a little and we were confident that no great harm would come to the older boys while Gemma and I looked after the younger ones. Inevitably, though, there was an 'incident'. Let's face it, it wouldn't be a Blaker trip without one. We were sitting in the lobby, Gemma reading one of their favourite Usborne touchy-feely books to Zoe and Edward, and me rocking the baby in my arms ('That's not my Bailey ... her mouth is too quiet'). Suddenly one of the hotel staff appeared, alerting us that our boys had been involved in an altercation in the hotel's manicured gardens, previously tended by Percy Thrower and his head gardener father. I rushed off to find the three boys looking shame-faced, while an angry-looking man, who I think was the current holder of that job, stood alongside them. I still don't know what happened as I couldn't get any sense out of the boys when it came to 'Rosegate'. They each did what they always do and said it was their brothers' fault rather than answering any of my questions. All I do know is, had Percy Thrower seen what my boys had done to these gardens, they would have caused him to cry even more than Les Ferdinand and Dennis Wise allegedly did 30 years earlier.

One might think after two failed attempts to enjoy a family holiday that we'd have left it there. Surely, though, by now you've realised we always do things the hard way. So a couple of years later we decided to see if it would be third time lucky by taking everyone off for another week away. And this time we were pulling out all the stops. We weren't going to Leicestershire; we weren't heading to Buckinghamshire; we were off to Bedfordshire. And before you scoff, this wasn't just anywhere in

Bedfordshire. We were packing everyone up and driving to Luton Airport, en route to Greece. What could possibly go wrong?

Amazingly, we managed to navigate our way through security without anyone being arrested and were feeling rather smug by the time we got to our gate. Unfortunately, this was when things started to go awry and we endured what has become known in our family, rather confusingly, as 'Gategate'.

It was probably a massive mistake to book easyJet, although flying with the budget airline has some remarkable parallels to travelling with my kids. The former is famous for selling cheap basic tickets, then making you cough up for everything from legroom to luggage, and my children have cleverly adapted this pricing policy for themselves. You buy them the plane ticket and think that's it, but then you've got to factor in all the extras. Drinks for everyone at the airport? £15. Food? That will be another £30. Then add magazines and colouring books to keep them quiet; money to play the arcade machines; an undisclosed fee that Adam is demanding to ensure his cooperation on the plane; and three charger cables from Currys to replace the ones that got broken on the way to the airport. Stelios would be very impressed.

Anyway, we arrived at the gate, and no sooner had we sat down than I heard our names read over the public address system. Shit! What have we done now?! It turned out there was an issue with our seating. We were too large a family to be together in one row, and yet the children were too young to sit without a responsible adult. I stared at the computer screen as they explained the problem, and it was like facing Deep Blue at chess.

Edward to King 4? He'd be too far from me. Gemma to Knight 2? Nope, because now Zoe would be left alone. Every move I proposed was impermissible, and even Garry Kasparov would have struggled to find a workable solution. The airline suggested we wait until everyone else was on board, and then we could see if anyone would be willing to move to sit with Adam, Ollie and Dylan.

The wait at the gate with my increasingly agitated children was bad enough, but the worst was yet to come. We trooped on board, where the cabin crew explained that the plane couldn't move until someone agreed to swap seats and sit beside my oldest three. The sound of tutting from the already seated passengers was so loud it briefly drowned out my boys' bickering. I don't think we'd have been any more unpopular had the steward announced we were members of ISIS and were hijacking the plane. Eventually, no doubt fearing the flight would never take off, a man in his 20s kindly volunteered and left his parents and sister to move five rows forward. He told me his name was Johnny Vine and I thanked him profusely, then introduced him to the boys. I explained to him that they didn't need to be entertained – that was the job of their screens – and I also gave the children a stern warning to behave. Like that's ever done me any good.

In fairness, this time they were well behaved. They were polite, personable and even chatty. Which was very good news for me, but very bad news for poor Johnny Vine, who hadn't appreciated what he'd signed up for when he sat down next to Dylan. He was already exhausted because he and his family were from Los Angeles and had recently endured an 11-hour flight to London. Now, they were off to Greece for a week, and he'd probably been hoping to shut his eyes and catch up with some sleep. It was never going to happen! Dylan heard his accent and was immediately excited.

'Where are you from?' he asked.

'LA,' replied Johnny.

Dylan cooed in approval. Everything he loved was American and most of it emanated from Hollywood. This was like an aspiring Muslim meeting a man who lives in Mecca. He might not be a prophet, but he's as close to one as you'll probably ever get.

'Do you like *The Simpsons?*' asked Dylan.

Johnny Vine really should have thought carefully before answering. The fool didn't realise the mistake he was about to make.

'Yes, I love it!'

Well, that was it. Forget any idea you have about sleeping, Johnny Vine, because you've now got over four hours of solid chat ahead of you.

Dylan's eyes lit up and he bombarded his new neighbour with every possible question on *The Simpsons*. Favourite episode, least favourite episode, most loved character, best cameo, funniest lines. At one point I overheard Dylan performing the entire sixth-season episode 'Homer the Great', including a very enthusiastic rendition of 'We Do (The Stonecutters' Song)'. Before getting on that flight, I think Johnny Vine had considered himself a fan of *The Simpsons*. Now he realised that he was nothing of the sort when compared with an obsessive eight-year-old with ASD.

Periodically, I got up from my seat to go back and check in on the boys. On each occasion I caught Dylan in mid-question.

'Who's your favourite *Spider-Man* villain?'

'Have you seen the *Star Wars Holiday Special?*'

'Do you live near Adam West?'

By the end of the flight Johnny Vine looked shell-shocked. The second we landed he barely waited for the seatbelt signs to be turned off. He was out of his seat and legging it to the doors to get away from his young friend as soon as possible. As he passed, he gave me a look of utter hatred for what I'd inflicted on him. 'Just be grateful you can get away from him. I have to listen to this the whole time!'

The story had a surprising coda. Extraordinarily, we arrived at our hotel and who should we see in reception but Johnny Vine and his family. Dylan noticed him first and excitedly called out, 'Johnny Vine!' He looked around at Dylan and it was like he'd seen a ghost. We barely saw Johnny Vine over the next seven days as I think he spent most of the week hiding in his room. On the rare occasions that he did venture down, he'd spot us – and a wide-eyed Dylan – and quickly reverse and head back to his room.

Bearing in mind how difficult vacations have been, we've unsurprisingly spent most school holidays staying at home and sticking to day trips. Not that these have been much easier. Only last week we took several of the children to Crystal Palace Park to see the dinosaur sculptures. Big mistake. It turns out Zoe has gone from being scared of dogs to being completely petrified of dogs, so a park full of canines was far from ideal. I had to immediately buy her an ice cream and sit her in the sand pit until she'd calmed down and stopped screaming. Even worse, Edward totally lost his rag because he said the dinosaurs weren't authentic enough. He spent the rest of the trip googling different dinosaurs to make his point. To be fair to Edward, the models are incorrect by modern standards, but even when I explained that they were produced in the 1850s and reflected the scientific understanding of the time, he was still no happier. There can't be many 12-year-olds whose foul mood is caused by a contempt for the Victorians and their substandard palaeontology.

Even when trips have been somewhat successful, I know they will always end the same way. Just before we head back to the car, I'll tell everyone we're about to leave and that there won't be a toilet available for two hours. 'Who needs a wee? Come on, it's your last chance! No one? All right, let's go.' Which of course means that within 25 minutes I'll be on the side of a busy A road helping everyone wee onto the hard shoulder. There's nothing like ending a family trip by choking on exhaust fumes as Edward tries to urinate while still watching *Return of the Jedi*. Pleasant it is not.

I still don't understand why our kids need to stare at a device for every second of a trip. When I was a child, my brother and I just looked out the window. If we were lucky we got one of those *I-Spy with David Bellamy* books, some of which were incredibly dull – *I-Spy Pond Life* – and others pretty much impossible – *I-Spy Dinosaurs*. Good luck completing that book on a drive from London to Bournemouth. Edward would have loved it in theory, but if he didn't enjoy the dinosaurs at Crystal Palace, imagine how disappointed he'd have been when he couldn't spot a Triceratops anywhere in the Home Counties.

I did once suggest they should put down their devices and look at the scenery. 'We need our screens,' answered

Dylan piously. 'If we look out the window, we might see something inappropriate.' As opposed to that super-child-friendly area known as the internet. Makes perfect sense.

I feel part of the issue with our children is that we've set the bar too high when it comes to trips. You know how they say overexposure to pornography can make people dissatisfied with their real-life partners? How porn addicts are on a never-ending search for novelty, and they can't get aroused by real-life sex anymore? Well, that's our children. When it comes to outings, I mean. They've been overexposed because Gemma and I have done so much fun stuff with them over the years – hidden beaches, battleships, tours of football stadia – a trip to the park is now too vanilla. We must come up with new and exotic ways to sate their jaded palate. And coincidentally, like many porn addicts' viewing preferences, our children's ideal outing involves food, dressing up and ritual humiliation.

There's one trip about which the children will always be excited, though unhappily it's also the most painful: the theme park. Adam, for one, loves anywhere with roll-ercoasters, especially those in which he gets wet. Put him in a log flume and he's as happy as a pig in shit.* And credit to Adam, he's a great person to have on a day at LEGOLAND or Chessington due to his diagnosis letter. Take this along to Guest Services and you'll receive an access pass that will allow you to skip the queues and turn what would be a downright miserable day into an

---

* If Disney ever builds a theme park for pigs, there should definitely be a ride called Shit, and I assume the porcine guests will love it.

only slightly miserable day. If possible, I always try to take Zoe too, since she's the only child with a Blue Badge, which is handy for parking close to the entry gates.

Unfortunately, these are the only small plus points. First, we need to decide what rides to go on, but with numerous *Zappas* consensus isn't easy to come by. The phrase goes, 'Two Jews, three opinions'. My family are 'eight Jews, 57 opinions', some of which are as helpful as suggesting rides at Chessington when we're having a day at LEGOLAND. Then it's lunch, but having children with multiple food-sensitives means no one can agree where to eat, so I end up buying 20 bags of crisps at an eye-watering £3.50 a packet.

Trips to a theme park also bring out my children's dubious social skills. I'm not sure whether it's the wait-ing in line – albeit for a tiny fraction of what most people suffer – or the excessive amounts of sugar they consume, but there's usually even more fighting and name-calling than normal. They argue about who's standing next to whom in the queue; who's in charge of holding the map; who's in charge of reading the map. And that's not to mention the literal fights about who sits next to whom in the car, what we listen to on the stereo and who should get to use the car's sole charger cable, while crisp and biscuit crumbs get thrown around the back seats. This may explain why I've spent 15 years driving the world's crappiest Toyota Previa. It wouldn't be a good idea to let our children loose on something that has any real value.* Who doesn't love a day out with everyone staring at you

---

* I genuinely realised one day that my wife's personalised numberplate is worth three times the car it's attached to.

and assuming you're the winners of a *Shameless* looka-like competition, followed by standing on an A road and getting them to wee on the hard shoulder?

A year ago Gemma and I took The Bailey and a friend to London Zoo, and it was the most incredible Damascene moment. Obviously being The Bailey, she didn't shut up at any point during this trip. She covered all the regular topics, from what nail varnish colour she's planning on painting to why the boys in their class aren't worthy of The Bailey's attention, girlfriend. But on that afternoon, I had an insight into what it would be like to have a more normal family. No one ran off screaming, frightening every other child at the zoo in the process. No one had a meltdown because his brother called him an abacus. No one refused to eat any food because it wasn't the right shade of white. It was just me, Gemma and two *Coldplays* – well, at least technically *Coldplays*, anyway – walking, chatting and looking at the animals. And it was amazing. Because if I hadn't realised it already, trips and holidays just weren't made for families like ours.

Say what you like about the pandemic – and a more fulsome discussion of that period is to come – but there was at least one big benefit of having to stay indoors, and that was not being able to do any family trips. As boring as it might have been staring at the four walls of our house, I feel like I've already done enough days out with the children for at least five lifetimes. Subsequently I relished having a year off, and if I ever felt a masochistic urge to recreate the experience I could always cram everyone into the parked car on our driveway and encourage them to watch a wildlife film on my iPad, while they sat in the back fighting over crisps.

OK, maybe us families with *Zappas* aren't designed for holidays, but here are a few tips to make your life easier.

1. Ignore social media

If you scroll through Facebook and Instagram, you'll no doubt see happy smiling families enjoying themselves on holidays. They aren't! Remember, they're probably hating it too, but putting on a brave face for the outside world.

2. If you do attempt a holiday, keep it simple

If you don't have to fly, then don't. You'll be reducing your carbon footprint and lowering your stress levels at the same time.

3. Arrange for extra help if possible

If you can afford to take someone along to help, that would be ideal. Zoe really needs one-to-one support, and if we won the lottery we'd certainly have someone accompany us on holiday just to assist with her. Admittedly that's a long shot, so if you wouldn't mind buying several copies of this book that would be appreciated.

4. Do what you can to keep them entertained

Travelling with *Zappas* is hard, so invest in treats to keep them occupied. Our boys loved the *Tintin* and *Asterix* series, so we always bought another couple of books for these occasions. The children were excited about the holidays as they knew they'd get new additions to their collection.

5. Enquire about accessibility

If you're going to a theme park – and may God have mercy on your soul – do what you can to get a diagnosis letter or other proof of your child's needs. You'll be able to skip the line, which if you have a child who finds queuing difficult is going to be invaluable. Likewise, investigate your child's eligibility to get a Blue Badge. We've really benefited from Zoe's because she finds walking very challenging, so being able to park close to our destination has been a genuine help. You may also qualify for a complimentary carer's ticket, which will help offset the preposterous cost of food and drink!

6. Think about siblings

If you have *Zappas*, they may not like leaving their familiar environment. This would be a shame for any *Coldplays* in the family, so try to take the latter away on their own for a few days if possible. Adam required so much of our attention, we always worried that Ollie might miss out. Hence, in 2013, I took him to Belgium for a weekend. He loved it and it was great to spend one-on-one time with him, especially in the years before he became an angry teenager.

7. Be positive because not everything is as it seems

You may think your family trips and holidays are a disaster, but your children's perception might be different. Researching this chapter, I asked my kids for their favourite memory from our many days out. Adam replied first. 'That time Dad threw up on the way to Chessington. That was amazing. Sick everywhere! And it was bright pink! You were completely covered in it!'

Dylan agreed. 'That was hilarious. And we wouldn't let you go home to get changed. You had to carry our stuff and go on all the rides, and everyone was looking at you like you were crazy!'

Even if you're having a bad time, it could be that you're still creating happy family memories when you least expected it. Happy for the children, anyway.

16

W IS FOR WAITING FOR THE BUS

So far we've covered the potential nightmare of getting your *Zappa* into the school of your choice; the challenges of keeping them happy once they've been accepted; and the torture of endless school meetings, with either biscuits or tissues. However, before you can even discover if your child was made for school or whether they think the normal rules apply to them, you must first transport them to the school gates.

Obviously, you could drive them but that may not be possible for several reasons. You might have other commitments that prevent you taking them every day; it may be impractical to set up a rota with other parents who won't know your child; and you may not want to be stuck in a car with a child droning on in a monotone voice about whether zombies exist because he saw a video on YouTube that says they are real and living in a village in South America but don't actually want to eat people and mostly keep themselves to themselves.

The good news is that your child might be entitled to free transport as part of their EHCP 'if they cannot walk to school because of their special educational needs and disabilities (SEND) or a mobility problem'.* The bad news is that if you're fortunate enough to get transport, you can add this to the interminable school meetings, exasperating hospital appointments and painful NHS interactions as sources of frustration in your life.

Of our children, Zoe is the one who is eligible for transport to and from school. This is arranged by the local council and so, in our case, it's a minibus organised by the London Borough of Barnet. Because she goes to a special school, nearly all the children have transport, with several minibuses collecting each child at their home in the morning and dropping them back in the evening. It's like those American school buses we see in TV shows such as *The Simpsons*, except the bus isn't yellow and the drivers are thankfully a lot safer than Otto.

Unfortunately, there are more than enough other aspects of transport that will cause you anxiety. As should be clear by now, the lives of parents of *Zappas* are often incredibly precarious. We muddle along, get help where we can and hope things fall in our favour. But it only takes one little thing to go wrong for everything to go tits up. And one of these little things is our children's transport, since we all rely on it to make our lives work. In our case, for everything else to happen – me and Gemma to be able to work, our other children to be taken to school – we need Zoe's bus to arrive by 8 a.m. As

---

* Evidently, this is the language of the UK Government website, since they use such long-winded terminology rather than the simple word *Zappas*.

anyone who's sat in rush-hour traffic knows, at that time of the morning, seconds count. Leaving five minutes late can add half an hour to your journey. If all goes to plan and she leaves on time then everything else should be OK, but if the bus is late we're in big trouble.

So while we're grateful that Zoe qualifies for free transport, the bus has become the bane of our life. The arrival time of 8 a.m. is purely notional. It has previously come at any point from 7.35 a.m. – when Zoe is still getting dressed – to as late as 11 a.m., by which point everyone else has missed the start of school by several hours. If I had a proper job, I really would be in shtuck.*

I must stress, it's a wonderful service 90 per cent of the time. The drivers we've had have been lovely, outgoing people, and become a large part of Zoe's life. There have been three permanent drivers in the past decade, all of them called Barry. I am yet to find out if this is a remarkable coincidence – a real million-to-one chance, I'd imagine – or whether it's like *Doctor Who*, and the driver has merely regenerated each time, while remaining the same person. Perhaps the bus is a TARDIS with a fixed chameleon circuit. It would certainly explain its rather random timekeeping. And impressively, the London Borough of Barnet cast a person of colour in the role of Barry a good three years before the BBC followed suit with Ncuti Gatwa. The bus also has an escort – no Adam, not that kind of escort – who is legally required to be on board to chaperone the children, and again, they've

---

* Don't think this book has written itself. I just meant I don't have a boss looking at his watch and saying sarcastic things like, 'Nice of you to join us.'

been charming. Our current escort is called Helen, and Zoe loves her. To continue the *Doctor Who* metaphor, the escort is like the companion; there in the background and always liable to change, but every bit as essential as their co-star.

The problem is that the very slightest thing will throw the bus off course and make it seriously delayed. It always reminds me of the excuses for Reggie Perrin's train being perpetually late.

'Signal failure at Vauxhall.'

'Defective bogey at Earlsfield.'

'Badger ate a junction box at New Malden.'

At least in *The Fall and Rise of Reginald Perrin* the train was never later than 22 minutes. We've waited literally hours for the bus on account of, among other things, traffic, bad weather, the driver being unwell, the escort being unwell, the driver oversleeping, a flat battery, a flat tyre, two flat tyres, broken windscreen wipers (whatever you do, please don't remind Zoe about 'Wipergate'!), another kid soiling themselves, a change of route due to a child moving house, Barnet losing the bus (how does that even happen?!) and Mars unexpectedly aligning with Jupiter.

Interestingly, while *some* of these could be attributed to acts of God – personally I refuse to believe in a God that's responsible for Barry oversleeping – there seems to be a particularly high probability of the bus being very late on the first day of a new term or following a bank holiday Monday. It's as if any break in the routine causes everyone involved to forget they were ever providing this service. They wake up on Tuesday morning after a long weekend, hungover, unable to remember their own name, and with a Mike Tyson-style tribal tattoo on their face, which they have no recollection getting.

As with the NHS, communication is not the local council's strong suit. We're never informed the bus is running late and must simply stare out the window, waiting for Barry to materialise. Alternatively, the council will cause absolute panic by announcing sudden changes that would, with no exaggeration, throw our lives into turmoil. A few weeks ago we received an email on a Sunday evening, mere hours before the start of term, to inform us that due to 'unforeseen circumstances' transport would be cancelled 'indefinitely'. No explanation was given, and naturally the parents' WhatsApp group was full of hysterical mums and dads who had no other means to get their children – some of whom are in wheelchairs and have extremely life-limiting disabilities – to school for the foreseeable future. It turned out that the escort was simply off sick, and Barnet couldn't find a replacement. It also became apparent that whoever wrote this email didn't understand the meaning of the word 'indefinitely', and caused great anxiety to a dozen families unnecessarily, because by the following day they'd located a stand-in escort and normal service was resumed. The relief among the parents was such that the anger over the 24 hours of stress Barnet had caused was almost instantly forgotten, although clearly not by me.

This may seem the most inconsequential chapter in this book. When it comes to raising children who have all manner of special needs and disabilities, surely there are bigger things to worry about than whether a bus is 15 minutes late?! What about whether your child will ever be able to live independently? Whether they will even live to be an adult? Or whether they will ever stop yammering on about videos they've watched online? And yes, of course, there are long-term concerns that outweigh our worries about the bus. But our daily wait is the perfect symbol of the everyday challenges of being a parent of kids with SEN. Because by and large, we don't think about the bigger worries as we'd drive ourselves mad. We'd live in a constant state of depression about the future. It is too upsetting to think your child may never get married, have a job or even see their 21st birthday. So we put all that to the back of our minds and try to live in the present. Get by as best we can. But for that to happen, we need all the moving parts of our life to work, and we can't do this alone. We rely on other people and services. And nothing is more emblematic of this than the wait for Zoe's bus. It's a daily reminder of how our lives are built on sand. That we have no control over them, and that any tiny break in the smallest link in the chain will mean one of us can't work or our other children will be late for school. A flat tyre on Barnet's bus can result in me not getting paid for a day. This is the reality for the parents of *Zappas*. All we can do is stare out the window and hope things will work out.

I wish I had some practical advice for other parents, but in this case I think I need to go a bit more zen (and the art of bus maintenance, at which Barnet don't seem to be very adept).

1. Accept this is your life

We depend massively on other people, even more than parents of *Coldplays*, so the smallest glitch can make our lives impossible. And that's just how it is, so reconcile yourself to the fact there will be times when it all goes wrong. SEN requires zen.

2. Put some contingencies in place

There will be days when the bus is late or your childcare doesn't arrive. At the very least, have some neighbours or friends you can call on. That won't be as easy as it would for parents of a *Coldplay*. We've struggled with this since children with SEN can't be left with just anyone. Zoe needs to know and trust someone. Meanwhile, we don't dislike anyone so much that we'd inflict our boys on them without the promise of payment. But if you can slowly develop these relationships over time, then when the shit hits the fan, hopefully your children will be comfortable and you'll have some help up your sleeve.

3. Get to know the other parents using transport

Form a WhatsApp group so when things go wrong, which they will, you'll be able to help each other out. When Zoe's bus was stopped 'indefinitely', she was given a lift to school by another parent, while a second parent brought her home. If nothing else, you can moan together and know you're not going through this alone.

4. Be on good terms with the bus driver and escort

In the same way that it's important to schmooze the consultant's secretary, have their direct number and keep them onside. Remember them at the end of term and Christmas. They do a tough job for little money, and your gratitude will be appreciated, so organise a gift with the other parents. If you have a good relationship, they'll hopefully let you know when they're running late, so you're not just looking out the window indefinitely (correct use of the word) and can make other plans.

5. Win the lottery

Then you can buy your own bus and pay for a chauffeur to drive it. Come to think of it, you've won millions, so get a limo instead. Just don't forget the other parents in your WhatsApp group, so spread the love and take their children too.

17

S IS FOR SPOUSE

If you're going to make it through the challenges of raising a child with SEN, then you need help. In our case it
would be fair to say no one has provided more support,
both emotional and practical, than our spouse. Of course,
I'm aware some of you reading this will be single parents
and trying to muddle along without any aid from a significant other, so I'll keep this chapter brief. Instead, I'd like
to hand over to my wife to finally say a few words herself.
Gemma, over to you.

*Thank you, Ashley, for giving me the opportunity to say
my piece.*

*It's definitely been a rollercoaster of a ride raising our
children over the past 18 years or so. There have been
some very trying moments, but we've been able to get
through them, and this has been in no small part due to
Ashley. He likes to play down his role, but when he says
I've done most of the work he's being falsely modest.*

*Did I really teach the children phonics on my own
while he sat watching football?! Even when he didn't
pull his weight on the homework front, it would only*

have been for a good reason, such as Liverpool playing a very important match.

Did I truly attend most of the meetings with the children's schools, while he sat in an office at the BBC writing jokes with Matt Lucas? Well, maybe sometimes, but even when Ashley wasn't available, he was there in spirit, which in many ways is more important than doing the meetings himself.

Have I genuinely done all the parenting while he's been on tour in the UK, Australia, South Africa or North America? Even when he's performed long runs Off-Broadway – for which, it should be said, he received incredible praise from the New York Times, New York Post and Wall Street Journal – Ashley has been constantly available on FaceTime, technically doing just as much of the hard graft, even though he couldn't literally do bath or bedtime. Surely everyone would agree, parenting from 3,500 miles away is even harder than doing it in person. Ashley's made himself available to listen to Dylan go on and on about things he's seen on YouTube, while also adjudicating 'Monstermunchgate', and for that alone he deserves great praise. What's more, he's done all this while bringing laughter to countless people across the globe, and that's an achievement that's not to be sniffed at!

Ashley is so humble that he'd never want to inflate his role, and naturally tries to be self-deprecating. But he's been every bit an equal in parenting our children, if not possibly doing slightly more of the work, now I come to think of it.

So, thank you, Ashley, on behalf of me and the children. We owe you so much.

Wow, thanks, Gemma. I must say, I really wasn't expecting that at all. I can't say I'm not touched. As she correctly pointed out, I don't like bigging myself up and was in two minds whether to even include this, but Gemma insisted. At the very least, let's move on quickly to the next chapter.

18

A IS FOR ADOPTION

Adoption is unquestionably a big topic that deserves its own book. However, it would be remiss not to touch on it seeing as there's a huge crossover between the issues of special needs and adoption. Many adopted children have additional challenges of some kind, even if they are hidden and only reveal themselves later. In 2017 an Adoption UK survey claimed that nearly half of all adopted children had recognised SEN or disabilities. Similarly, a 2023 survey found that a third of all Blaker children with a diagnosis were adopted, so this is a subject close to my heart.

The abundance of extra needs among adoptees is understandable when one considers the reasons children may find themselves adopted to begin with. A whopping and frankly tragic 75 per cent come from a background of abuse, trauma and neglect, all of which can lead to a plethora of issues such as developmental delay, attachment disorders and sensory processing difficulties. There's a higher incidence of foetal alcohol spectrum disorders. And this is before we get to other special needs or disabilities that may have contributed to children either being placed into care or, in some cases, being given up for adoption. But I'm not here to frighten you. Please don't read this and be put off from adopting. It is without doubt one of the most rewarding things we've ever done and choosing a child with Down syndrome gave me a completely different perspective on SEN in general. But before I tell you why, let me do my best Max Bygraves impression because 'I wanna tell you a story'.*

My tale starts in the summer of 2010. Back then Donald Trump was just that orange man from the American version of *The Apprentice*; a Remainer was something in the toilet that requires a plunger; and self-isolation was an activity teenage boys did on their own, unless they went to boarding school, in which case they did it all together. What simple times. Well, simple for most people, but certainly not for me and Gemma because by then we already had four boys aged six, five, three and a baby barely two months old. And remember, these weren't just any children: these were Blakers. To recap, Adam had already been diagnosed with autism; Dylan was three years away from being diagnosed with autism; Ollie was eight years away from being diagnosed as the world's angriest pre-teen in history; and Edward wasn't even in a night-time routine, though I'm sure he was already dreaming about nothing except dinosaurs and LEGO.

So when I was flipping through the adverts in a local newspaper one evening I should have been on the

---

* One for the kids there!

lookout for nannies and childminders for the kids, or at the very least a drug dealer for me and Gemma. However, the ad that drew my attention was from the London Borough of Hackney. It had the headline:

> Opt to Adopt. Zoe is 'simply beautiful'. Could you be the family for her?

At this point, any sane person would have stopped reading and headed straight for the sudoku. Possibly turned to the section on home baking to get a ten-year head start with their lockdown sourdough. Because 'Could you be the family for her?' shouldn't have been the toughest question in the world to answer. As a quiz question, it was hardly up there with 'What is the shortest of Shakespeare's plays?' since without even thinking, the correct response was obviously NO WAY IN HELL. By a funny coincidence, our attempts to build a normal family home had been *The Comedy of Errors*.

Besides, the pedant in me was immediately put off by the use of a pull quote – 'simply beautiful' – without any source. Who was saying this exactly? If only this kind of thing was allowed in publishing, I'd make sure this book was covered in similarly unverifiable praise: 'Utter genius', 'I couldn't put it down,' 'Does for raising children with SEN what *Fifty Shades of Grey* did for S&M'.

Yet despite all of this, and against my better judgement, I read on …

> Zoe is a happy and loving little girl. She is eating solids and has a good routine. She is sleeping twice in the day and sleeps all night.

Well, at least that sounded encouraging.

> Zoe is a child with Down syndrome.

Ah. And suddenly alarm bells were ringing. Surely now was the time to put the paper away and turn on the TV instead.

> Zoe is attending physiotherapy every second week due to her low muscle tone. She is doing extremely well and can sit up on her own.

Interesting to see that they acknowledged Zoe had physio once a fortnight, but conveniently forgot to mention the other 28 appointments each month.

> Zoe has a slight hearing loss, however it is not causing her any major problems.

'It will cause *you* major problems because you'll be the poor sod doing the ENT and audiology visits, but we'll also keep schtum about that for now!'

> Her foster carer is teaching her Makaton sign language to encourage her speech and language development to which she is responding well. The prospective adopters would also need to be able to continue teaching Zoe Makaton.

As luck would have it, we had the resources from when we briefly considering teaching Adam, but this felt like a massive undertaking. For a start, I'd have to find the books, which had been stored somewhere in the loft alongside our suitcases.

The advert ended with a request for potential adopters who would be patient (not my best quality), compassionate (a virtue which, if I ever had it, was already being tested to the limit), humble (now *that* I'd say I'm very good at), and who'd be able to provide a stable, nurturing family. Well, let's just say if you'd come to our home in 2010 I doubt you'd have thought we were serious candidates. And yet somehow, amazingly, perhaps even miraculously, this adoption happened. Independently, Gemma and I had both seen this advert for a family to adopt a 12-month-old girl with Down syndrome and thought we could do it. This despite possessing almost none of the credentials the advert requested. Then again, is job suitability ever really that important? The government's only qualification for PPE contracts was living near Matt Hancock, and that worked out fine.

The obvious question is why we even considered it, bearing in mind our already frantic homelife. And the honest answer is I genuinely have no idea. You know how people sometimes explain criminal acts as having been the result of a 'moment of madness'. 'I've never stolen pic 'n' mix sweets before, I don't know what came over me!' 'I've never parked in a parent and child bay before, I don't know what came over me!' 'I've never put on a fur hat with horns and broken into the US Senate Chamber before, I don't know what came over me!'

I'm not sure if this was madness, naivety or bravery, but whatever it was, it simultaneously came over both of us. Although if you're currently thinking we must be saints, I will admit it was more Gemma than me. I think I'd merely been watching too much of *The Jeremy Kyle Show* and wanted to be able to say I also had children from two different mothers.

After the briefest of conversations between us, I got in touch with Hackney's Children and Families Service department, and they arranged a home visit from a social worker. Sadly, they weren't interested in taking any of our kids into care and only wanted to discuss us adopting Zoe. I'd hoped for a part-exchange for my eldest son at the very least, but they wouldn't hear of it. Nonetheless, barely a week later they were in our house and the ball was rolling.

The first thing we discovered is that the process of approval is extremely full-on and will usually take nine months. At first I assumed this period was chosen purposely to mirror pregnancy, perhaps as a kindness to those that couldn't have children and would appreciate the symmetry. My cynical mind also figured they'd make adopters wait nine months to ensure no one used this as a short cut to parenthood. Of course, my theory was nonsense because these nine months are just the beginning of the process, and can be followed by months or even years of waiting to be matched with a child, which has its own separate assessment procedure. The reason this initial part of the journey lasts nine months is simply because the wheels move unbearably and, to my eyes, unnecessarily slowly.

Social services would argue the time is needed to ensure that children – moreover, often the most vulnerable of children – are not placed at risk by being entrusted

with people who are unsuitable or in some way danger-
ous. And obviously, children's safety must always be
paramount. However, it's galling to think two teenagers
could have drunken sex this evening and create a baby
with no adjudication regarding their suitability to be
parents. For adopters the bar is incredibly high, while for
everyone else the bar is non-existent. OK, rant over. I'll
just say, if you get off on unnecessary bureaucracy,
applying to adopt could be the hobby for you.

Hackney promised to investigate every aspect of our
life including our relationship, finances, personalities
and family, though thankfully not my internet history.
Still, there were plenty of other embarrassments ahead.
To prove we could afford to adopt Zoe, we had to hand
over bank statements, pay slips and annual accounts,
and complete a budget outlining our monthly outgoings.
It wasn't easy to explain why I was spending half our
money on comics, football tickets and haemorrhoid
cream.

Even more humiliating was when we were required to
fill in a diagram that would hopefully show what a big
support network we could rely on. I'm afraid to say this
involved us stretching the truth a little about how popular we were. Our form included claims like, 'I have many
friends from the local synagogue,' which translated
meant, 'I know some people from the local synagogue,
who I regularly use for comic material.' Likewise, the
claim, 'We are very close to our neighbours the Harleys,'
which really meant, 'We live physically close to our
neighbours the Harleys, but they don't talk to us since I
had a lawyer send them a cease and desist letter for
running an illegal car park on their driveway.'

By far the worst aspect of the process was having meeting after meeting with our social worker Clare, whose job it was to assess us via all manner of increasingly intrusive and bafflingly abstruse enquiries. Much of it was very politically correct, with questions such as, 'What is your view of Britain as a multi-racial society?' and 'Do you have any LGBTQ friends?' At least that one was easy to answer since at the time I worked in television. It would be best to find a different industry if you have a problem with homosexuals. Or Jews. Or especially with homosexual Jews.

Unfortunately these kinds of questions aren't good for a cynic like me, and I'd often take them less seriously than I should have done. When asked, 'Have you ever read a book or seen a film that was about adoption?' I replied, 'How about *The Omen*?' I was hoping Clare would laugh. Instead, she straight-batted this away, saying she hadn't seen it and asking how the adoption worked out. Two can play at that game. I answered with as impassive a face as possible, 'Not great. He turned out to be the son of the devil, born of a jackal, the final manifestation of the antichrist on Earth.' The only other film I could think of that featured adoption was *Star Wars*, which teaches us that if siblings are ever adopted, it's best to keep them together, otherwise maybe one day they'll make out with each other.

The biggest issue for me was that most of the hypothetical questions, usually aimed at childless candidates, involved trying to find out what kind of parents we'd be if we ever had kids. They didn't acknowledge that we had made four already and had developed our own, albeit flawed, parenting style. Clare would ask things like, 'If a child's favourite cereal ran out, what do you think you would do?' with such difficult multiple-choice answers as:

    A. Go to the shops and buy them the cereal.
    B. Give them dog food.
    C. Make them go hungry.

Irritatingly, she didn't give the option of what we'd really do:

    D. Tell them we've been given a secret new type of Coco Pops with the shape, style and taste of Shredded Wheat.

Even as teenagers, I'm pretty sure my boys would fall for that.

The investigation went on and on, and the questions became more and more esoteric. We were sent a 12-page form with over 200 questions, which was so in-depth it took more than a week to complete. It mostly focused on our own childhoods, with such lines as:

All families have secrets. Please share any secrets that affected you during your upbringing.

This felt like the kind of gnomic question one would find in the exam for a fellowship at All Souls College, Oxford. Was this not a trick question? Surely if I tell you a secret, then it's no longer a secret?

There were also many intrusive questions about our sex life such as:

> Who taught you about sex or increased your knowledge/awareness?

In my case, Paul Raymond, obviously.

> What adjustments have you had to make in your sexual relationship?

At this time, we had four boys aged six and below, including a baby yet to be in a routine. What adjustments do you think we've had to make?!

> How do you deal with differences in your sexual needs?

As I said, I was relieved they didn't want to see my internet history.

Perhaps a reader will tell me why these questions were so important, but it was hard not to feel the social workers were taking a rather prurient interest in our personal lives.

Most extraordinarily, one day Clare phoned me in a total panic. She said the adoption panel were meeting in a few days and she'd just realised there was a big hole in her report about us. I wondered what it could be. Was it to do with our financial stability? Did they need to know more about our time commitments? Was it to find out if I ever did get that threesome? Nope, she wanted to know, when I was in primary school, did I get invited to many birthday parties. I'm not making this up. For some reason, the massive hole the social worker was concerned about was whether 30 years ago I'd eaten enough jelly. To this day I'm completely clueless as to what she'd hoped to glean from the answer. Perhaps when adopting a child, one needs to remember the lessons one learnt from playing Musical Statues and Pass the Parcel. Honestly, your guess is as good as mine.

The final stage of the process was a very thorough medical examination. I briefly sweated over the potential embarrassment of being the first person to be turned down as an adopter on the grounds of athlete's foot and piles. Social services also went to the police to check whether we had a criminal record, and again I was slightly worried, but was relieved when I realised it was only a check on me and Gemma and not our sons. Although, even if they were included, causing actual bodily harm in a soft-play ball pool is a tough crime to pin on a six-year-old. Plus, the non-verbal are notoriously hard to crack under questioning.

As we edged closer to being approved, we felt sufficiently confident to finally tell our boys what was happening, using a book given to us by our social worker called *Nutmeg Gets Adopted*. It's about a small red squirrel called Nutmeg whose mother isn't able to look after him and his younger siblings, and so is adopted by a family of badgers. At first it sounded far-fetched, but I guess it could happen. Obviously, it would depend on how many birthday parties the badgers had been to when they were cubs, and how they resolved the differences in their sexual needs. Yet I'm still not convinced it's an ideal match. Squirrels are herbivores, while badgers eat mostly earthworms and other invertebrates. I've got to be honest, if you're so concerned that we wouldn't give a child their favourite cereal, I don't know why you'd place a squirrel with badgers. The judge in this story is an owl, and I can only think that being a nocturnal animal, the day he signed off on this case he was half-asleep.

It's a very sweet book but is aimed at 'normal' children. Sadly, that's definitely not my boys, who took this story to mean that we were literally adopting a squirrel. They were genuinely baffled the day they were introduced to a little girl with Down syndrome, rather than the new rodent member of the family. The less said about 'Squirrelgate' the better.

The final step, and by far the hardest, was letting my parents in our plans. Of all the challenging conversations you can have with your family – 'I need to tell you, I'm gay!'; 'I need to tell you, we're getting divorced!'; 'I need to tell you, I'm marrying an American actress, moving to California and will cause you even more grief than Uncle Andrew!' – they are nothing compared with, 'I need to tell you, we've decided our four crazy boys aren't enough work, and we want to add a two-year-old with Down syndrome to see if this will finally break us.' This was akin to standing in front of the fire at Notre-Dame and thinking, let's see if it helps to lob in a petrol bomb.

As difficult as it would have been to tell any set of parents, it was especially hard telling mine because, God bless 'em, they aren't the most adventurous people. A big change for them is one night watching *EastEnders* before *Coronation Street*. We dreaded their reaction, and so while we had the courage to adopt Zoe, we chickened out of informing my parents face to face and sent an email instead. Even worse, to buy us a bit more time we did it late at night after they'd gone to sleep. So, if you were going to nominate us for an award for bravery, you might want to think again. It would be like Ernest Shackleton being sufficiently heroic to head to the Antarctic but not willing to first tell his mum.

It was nearly a week until we heard from my parents, but having had six days to compose themselves, they just about concealed their opinion that we were certifiably insane. And in fairness, they did wish us luck and say they'd view Zoe like any of our other children. Now that might just have meant they'd look at her and think, 'She can't possibly be related to us,' because I imagine that's what they thought when they saw our boys. Although in the case of Zoe, this would finally be true.

Anyway, with my parents on board and all the reports completed, we were pretty much there. Finally, after many months of meetings and assessments, the big day came when we were all introduced to Zoe. The boys wondered who this girl was when they were expecting a squirrel; I prayed that she hadn't been born of a jackal; and we all started to get to know each other. Answering all the social worker's questions had been hard enough, but now the real work began. For what happened next, just read on.

19

L IS FOR LOVE
LIKE NO OTHER

In the 12 years since Zoe moved into our home many people have asked me questions about it. I've heard them all: 'What prompted you to do it?'; 'Do you think she knows she's adopted?'; 'Why didn't we get a squirrel when that's what you promised us?' But the question I've been asked more than all the others combined is, 'Are you able to love Zoe as much as your other children?' And the honest answer, I'm ashamed to say, is no. I love her a lot more.

On reading this, I imagine my boys and The Bailey will be going crazy, but please, let me explain. You see, I truly believe that the love one has for an adopted child is so great, that it's possibly among the purest forms of love there is. And even more so when that adopted child has special needs.

Obviously, I love all my children; most of the time anyway. All parents love their children. I'm sure even Mr and Mrs Hopkins look at Katie and think, 'Ah, we did well there.' Yet if we parents are being sincere, there's a certain degree of narcissism involved. Our children are an extension of us, preserve a part of us in the world and usually even look like us, which has been very bad luck for my sons. They aren't bald yet, but as I keep reminding them, they probably have only a decade or so to enjoy their hair. The same goes for their pain-free feet and anus.

However, when it comes to Zoe, there can't be any degree of narcissism involved because she shares none of our genes. And I can tell this because as a result of not being biologically mine, she's by far and away the most impressive member of the Blaker household. No offence if you're reading this, boys. Zoe will frequently say, 'I love you, Daddy; I love you, Mummy.' Meanwhile, Ollie communicates via scribbled notes left on the kitchen counter, which at their most polite will read, 'Buy a new charger cable or I'll kill you.' Even if you're making death threats, you could still say please! Zoe's school can't praise her enough, while barely a day goes by without a phone call from one of the boys' schools to tell us, 'There's been an incident.' Zoe goes to bed when we ask her. In contrast, our boys each enter full-on barrister mode as they argue for 20 more minutes of *Grand Theft Auto*, which will frequently involve invoking the Magna Carta.*

My love for Zoe is a special love because it's not influenced by the fact that she's biologically related to me. It's true that your spouse isn't going to be related to you either, unless you're like Queen Elizabeth II and married your cousin. But even assuming you didn't wed a family member, the love you have for your husband or wife isn't

---

* For the avoidance of doubt, that was a joke. If it were true, it would mean they'd been paying attention in their history lessons.

quite as special because it's in many ways conditional. In our case, we've an unwritten contract that Gemma will cook all the food and I promise to never go near her with my infected feet.

Conversely, with Zoe there are no conditions at all, because due to her special needs she can't give much back. And that will probably never change. In the future she won't be capable of caring for us in our old age. On the contrary, we'll be looking after her. At least when my other children were babies, I wiped their soiled bottoms cheered by the fact that one day the roles will be reversed and they'll have to do the same for me. When my boys annoy me, I look forward to inflicting as much discomfort on them in the future as possible. That would be fitting penance for 'Pubesgate'.*

Zoe gives back with a smile, a kiss and a cuddle, but she's sometimes too grumpy to even give that. And yet I still love her. I love her despite the fact we aren't biologically related, and despite the fact she isn't able to give much in return. This love isn't familial; it isn't conditional; it is surely the purest love there is. I will admit I do have an enormous love for Jürgen Klopp, to whom I'm also unrelated, at least to the best of my knowledge. I think the Liverpool manager is probably the only man in the world for whom I'd happily go gay. But if I'm honest, this love is based on the condition that he wins us trophies, so I love Zoe even more.

We love Zoe simply because of who she is. Because like everyone with special needs, she teaches us the

---

* I won't embarrass the culprit, nor will I go into details in case you're eating a meal.

inherent value in people. That your worth isn't defined by what you do, or what you achieve, or how many followers you have on Instagram.* Zoe shows us that people have value simply because they exist, and because this is how God, the universe, the Midi-chlorians or whatever it was, created them.

In fact, if I ever had doubts that a higher power runs the world, our adoption of Zoe was the final proof I needed. There simply must be, because there's no other explanation as to how this family, with four boys who are basically a distillation of all my wife's and my worst character traits, could possibly have been approved adopters. No one in their right mind would have handed this sweet girl to us to look after. The fact this was the decision of social services and a judge, who was neither an owl nor any other somnambulant nocturnal creature, is concrete evidence that God runs the universe according to His own mysterious plan. You can shake your head all you like, but if you saw what our family looked like in 2010, even Richard Dawkins would become a believer.

The second-most asked question in relation to Zoe – well, after all the ones from social services about our sex life – is, 'Have there been any downsides to adopting her?' The flippant response to which is yes, answering all the questions from social services about our sex life. But for once, let me answer more seriously. This chapter isn't intended as an advert for Adoption UK, so I'm happy to admit that it's come with some huge challenges.

---

* Although if you wish to follow, please do so by searching for @TheAshleyBlaker. I only have a modest number of followers, but at least I do have a verified blue checkmark.

For one, it has introduced the concept of adoption to our household. Strictly speaking that wasn't Zoe, it was Nutmeg the squirrel. But either way, the kids were now aware that children could potentially be raised by another family, and arguments suddenly had an all-new dimension.

'Adam's putting Coco Pops in my ear! Have him adopted!'

'Bailey ate my chocolate. Have her adopted!'

'Dylan took my charger cable. Have him adopted!'

Typically, Adam still doesn't get it and has been heard complaining, 'Zoe looked at me! Have her adopted!' Gemma or I are then required to remind him that Zoe has been already. Unfortunately, parents can't get themselves adopted. Trust me, I've tried.

However, a bigger issue we've experienced is what I believe to be the greatest taboo around adoption. Basically, that no matter what happens, however difficult your child may end up, you can never complain because there will always be someone, not least my mother, to say, 'Well, no one you asked to adopt!' To clarify, she only says that to us. If you were thinking of adopting, don't worry, my mum won't be turning up at your house to say no one asked you to do this. But I guarantee you, someone else will. And this drives me mad, because unless I didn't read the small print, when we signed the adoption papers it didn't say, 'Thou shalt never complain about this child, because you chose her so shut up and get on with it.'

I honestly don't understand this. No one would say to struggling parents who had previously suffered years of infertility, 'Well, no one asked you to have IVF.' I can't think of any other circumstance where people are so unsupportive. You wouldn't call the AA when you'd broken down on the M1 if you thought they'd reply, 'Well, no one asked you to buy a Renault!'

It's true, no one asked us to adopt Zoe, but so what? It doesn't make parenting her any less arduous. And Zoe, bless her, isn't easy. Getting her dressed in the morning is a massive operation that frequently resembles a particularly challenging game of Twister. For breakfast she wants cornflakes, but almost all of them end up on the floor, and while eating the remaining 5 per cent she takes her shoes off 15 times. Eventually she settles down to watch her iPad, but for some reason she only likes watching YouTube videos of *Peppa Pig* dubbed into Gujarati. Maybe she was a Hindu in a former life, although I can't imagine what sin she'd have committed to be punished by being reincarnated as a Blaker. We've had full-blown tantrums simply because she could only find *Peppa Pig* in Arabic. Zoe clearly wasn't a Muslim in a former life, although it would explain why she keeps taking her shoes off. But I can't complain about this to anyone. Obviously, I just moaned to you, but I imagine you're now shouting at the page, 'Well, no one asked you to adopt her!' If it's difficult, we must suck it up; in the case of her cereal, literally.

And as I said, Zoe is probably the crowning achievement and joy of our family. But even this is problematic, because it means everything that's virtuous about us was provided by a set of genes other than mine and Gemma's. It's not a great feeling when you realise all your daughter's good qualities were inherited from her birth parents. Or possibly just the result of her past life in India. Most likely they were instilled by her amazing foster parents,

Laura and Ian, with whom she lived until she was two and a half. All we've done is ruin that by giving her an iPad and getting her addicted to *Peppa Pig* in Gujarati. At least I suppose that means we've introduced her to a second language.

I will say, there's something to be said for adopting a child who's already been living with a foster family for two years, because it's one of the cliches of parenting that kids don't come with an instruction manual. But Zoe did! A 25-page instruction manual that covered everything from what song needs to be sung at bedtime to all the things she's scared of: the dark, clowns, shadows, flies, spiders, dogs, cats, windscreen wipers, umbrellas and flowers. Good luck taking her to the park. It even listed what food she liked at each juncture of the day – tuna and steamed vegetables?! – and sadly, I can only put her subsequent stroppiness and sugar addiction down to becoming a Blaker.

This is how parenting should always be. No more wondering whether your child needs an afternoon nap; page six of the instruction manual says she goes to bed at two o'clock with the light off and the door shut. It was even better than buying a computer, because if we had any issues, Laura and Ian offered phone support 24/7. What's more, they never put us on hold, weren't based in Bangladesh, and never once suggested turning her off and on again. This side of adoption is so incredible that when we had our next child I did wonder if we could deposit her with Laura and Ian for a few years. Let them do all the sleepless nights, get Bailey into a good routine and we'll pick her up when she's toilet trained. You do the hard graft; we'll take all the credit.

So that's our story of adoption. It's a very unusual case, not least because we had four sons already. But despite the huge challenges, we are all one (occasionally) happy family. Moreover, there's something incredibly special knowing your child was a choice. It's an amazing privilege to be able to turn to your child, look them in the eye and say, 'We chose *you*.' This child wasn't the result of us having too many glasses of wine one Friday evening. Sorry, Adam. They were a choice, and even more so when they have Down syndrome.

Having a child is a bit of a lottery. You can be lucky and have a baby who'll go on to achieve everything you dream for them; get a great job, make a fortune, and buy you a new house and a nice car, so you no longer need to drive around in an old Toyota Previa. Or you can have my children, who are the reason we have that old Previa, because I can't risk them destroying a car that's worth more than £50. But all this is irrelevant when it comes to Zoe. We can look at her and say, 'We chose you. Not for the glory you'll bring us, or the exam results, or the prestigious university you'll attend. Simply because we take pleasure in your existence and want nothing more than to see you grow and cheer you on as you reach your potential. We chose you exactly the way you are and the way you'll always be. We chose you because you have worth, and we want to love you.'

It's no understatement to say that adopting a child with special needs gives you a completely different perspective. Over the years I've chatted with many parents of *Zappas* about their experiences, and in a great number of cases there's been a prevailing sadness. These mums and dads had thought they were going to have a regular child, and then the tables were turned and they had a boy or girl with special needs. They were expecting to go to Washington, DC, and ended up in Washington, Tyne and Wear. At this point they went through various stages of shock and grief, and had serious fears about their child's future. But while this is all understandable, and are feelings to which we can relate, this just isn't our experience with Zoe. We adopted her. We knew she had Down syndrome. This wasn't a tragedy that happened to us, this was our choice. It was a choice taken with great joy and excitement, and was the most rewarding choice we've ever made, because having Zoe in our life is such a remarkable blessing.* And the truth is, over 12 years on, it's like Zoe has always been here and I've completely forgotten there was a time when this wonderful girl wasn't my own daughter. On the contrary, I tell strangers who meet us that my wild children are all adopted. Except for Zoe; she's my one biological child.

---

* And in case you're reading this, yes, the rest of you are also a blessing. Talk about having a chip on your shoulder!

20

C IS FOR
CELEBRATIONS

Just in case you wondered, this chapter is not about chocolate. As a matter of fact, someone did once buy us a tub of Mars Celebrations, and it led to a horrific incident memorialised as 'Celebrationsgate'.* No, this chapter is about celebrating family occasions, which, if you have a *Zappa*, may well look rather different than you'd imagined.

More specifically, it's about Adam's *bar mitzvah*. For those unaware, a *bar mitzvah* is a Jewish coming of age ceremony, held when a boy turns 13. There's a similar ritual for females called a *bat mitzvah*, which is celebrated when a Jewish girl becomes 12, presumably because they mature a year before boys, unless we're comparing them with my sons, in which case it's probably more like 20 years.

---

* 'Celebrationsgate' was much more traumatic than the previous 'CadburyHeroesgate', although possibly not in the same league as the truly harrowing 'QualityStreetgate'.

According to Jewish law, this is the age at which a child is held liable for their own actions, and parents are no longer responsible for their son's or daughter's deeds. And if you've seen Adam misbehaving over the past five years, please keep this in mind. Gemma and I are in no way accountable anymore, and if you don't believe me I can put you in touch with a rabbi. More practically, a *bar* or *bat mitzvah* involves the child doing something in synagogue followed by a big party. Parents often put themselves in debt celebrating the occasion. My own *bar mitzvah* in February 1988 was a grotesque black-tie event at a hotel in Belgravia that had little to do with me – frankly, I might as well have not been present – and all about my parents impressing their family and friends.

Modern parties often involve a four-course dinner, a disco, live music, photo booths, scantily clad waitresses pouring cocktails and people I now understand are called motivators. These are almost always Afro-Caribbean men, whose job it is to come on the dancefloor and show everyone how to dance and have a good time. I must be frank and say it always makes me feel a little uncomfortable. It's like we're saying, 'Us Jews, we're accountants and lawyers; we're not very good at letting our hair down. Can you please come along and show us how to really "get down", as I believe you'd say?' That said, maybe it works the other way too. I'd love to think if you go to a black family's wedding, that at some point in the evening they bring out an old rabbi to totally ruin the party.

Regardless of how it ends up looking, it's a rare Jewish parent – OK, let's adhere to the stereotypes and make that a rare Jewish mother – who doesn't sit with a new-born child in her arms and dream about their *bar* or *bat mitzvah*. It's the culmination of 12 or 13 years of parental care, a moment of intense pride as her offspring takes their place as a Jewish adult. Yes, it's a chance to impress other people, and there are many who make parties purely to keep up with the Cohens, but it's genuinely a deeply meaningful celebration.

We'd looked forward to our eldest son's *bar mitzvah* since Adam's birth in July 2004. The date in 2017 was marked in our calendars and a countdown was started. But with six months to go before the big day, it became apparent there was a problem. Adam absolutely, unequivocally refused to attend his own *bar mitzvah*. Forget the eponymous 'Bar Mitzvah Boy' in Jack Rosenthal's legendary *Play for Today*; he merely ran away from the synagogue mid-service. Adam wasn't even willing to go that far. He wouldn't learn any of the texts required, and with typical Blaker belligerence he declined to attend synagogue at all. The only time I could get Adam to come along was when I bribed him with the offer of as many energy drinks as he could stomach. Considering Red Bull is meant to give you wings, I suppose we might have hoped for angelic behaviour. Sadly, Adam acted so badly that he'd have been more welcome in synagogue were he Mel Gibson, eating a bacon sandwich, while listening to an album by Kanye West. We'd already suffered the ignominy of Adam refusing to wear smart clothes and being the sole congregant in a Liverpool shirt. It isn't a good look to turn up to synagogue in a football top, and even more so if it's not Tottenham Hotspur's.

I found it hard to adjust from what I'd imagined our son's *bar mitzvah* would look like to the reality, but this was nothing compared with poor Gemma. In her fantasies she was the glamorous mother in a long, flowing dress, for some reason bearing an uncanny resemblance to Gisele Bündchen. It wasn't because she had a desire to be the centre of attention. That isn't Gemma at all. It was because, as you'll be aware by now, the previous 13 years raising this autistic boy had been a struggle, to say the least. In fact, the word 'struggle' doesn't really do it justice. So why shouldn't Gemma have had one day of validation? After this traumatic journey, a *bar mitzvah* celebration in which she could bask would have been some small payback for all the years of assessments, specialist teachers, social workers, speech therapists, humiliations, sleepless nights, lawyers, cancelled social arrangements, sibling arguments and relationship trauma, not to mention 'Butchergate', 'Footgate' and 'Escortgate'. This *bar mitzvah* would make it all worthwhile.

'Talk to him,' she hissed at me as we perched outside Adam's room, two months away and still with nothing booked.

I wasn't particularly keen, especially as I was still recovering from a discussion about the Facts of Life that didn't go quite as planned. 'Please don't make me do another big talk.'

'But I'm getting nowhere!' Gemma protested. 'I need this *bar mitzvah*! I need to feel like we're a successful, functioning, normal family.'

At this moment, as if on cue, Dylan passed us on the stairs. 'I just had some delicious wallpaper for supper,' he told us. 'Why didn't you tell me that stuff tastes so good?'

I looked at her pityingly. 'Yes, Gemma. A successful, functioning, *normal* family.'

Adam emerged from his room, possibly to find out what the noise was or alternatively to sample the wallpaper before it was all gone.* I seized the bull by the horns.

'You're having a *bar mitzvah*,' I told him. 'With a hall, and a band, and a caterer, and me and mummy losing 20 lbs each, and you're turning up, and you will comply and behave and not be naked, and you're going to give a speech about how you owe everything to us, but mainly to your mum. And that's final.'

Adam started to cry, and Gemma immediately put her arm around him. 'Now look what you've done,' she said. That's gratitude for you!

I hate the fact that I brought Adam to tears. I also hate the fact that it only happened in a last-ditch attempt to rescue Gemma's Gisele Bündchen fantasy. But we needed this confrontation to come to our senses and realise that we'd collided with a boundary. In this case, it was the boundary between what we wanted and what we were actually getting. We – well, more Gemma if I'm being honest – had convinced ourselves that we needed this *bar mitzvah* to be happy. We required it to help bury the ghosts of the childhood we felt Adam owed us. After everything we'd given up, this seemed like one broken dream too many. But Adam's reaction showed us we had a simple choice: to either battle reality or practise acceptance. Maybe it wasn't quite as instantaneous as that, and there may have been some sulking and brooding over the following days, again, more Gemma here than me.

---

* Unfortunately, space dictates that I can't elaborate further on 'Wallpapergate'.

Crucially, though, we realised there was an alternative to feeling bad. That rather than fighting, crying and making everyone miserable, we could take a different path.

We didn't mention the B-word for another fortnight. It was then, now with just six weeks to go and peer pressure from all the *bar mitzvahs* in Adam's class overwhelming for Gemma and me, that we once again found ourselves outside the door of his bedroom. However, this time, we'd altered our approach.

'What do *you* want to do for your *bar mitzvah*?' Gemma asked him, just about managing to keep the grudging tone out of her voice.

He shrugged. 'Have a party with my friends. Order pizza. Play video games.'

Which was fine, because we'd finally accepted that it wasn't about us. We'd spent years fighting with schools to get them to make 'reasonable adjustments', and it was now time for us to do the same. Besides, I'd hated my *bar mitzvah* because I felt like the least important person there. Even more reason, then, to learn from the past and do the opposite; to make a *bar mitzvah* at which our precious son would feel comfortable and that he'd enjoy.

We abandoned the ceremonial aspect in a synagogue altogether and focused entirely on the evening event. He asked for a party with his friends involving pizza and video games, so that was exactly what we gave him. We placed an order for thirty pizzas. We cleared out the furniture and Edward's LEGO from the front room – best not to dwell on the drama that was 'LEGODeathStargate' – and produced invitations online. In a sole nod to more extravagant *bar mitzvah* parties, we hired a photo booth, which proved remarkably popular with all my children.

Who'd have thought that kids who normally require serious inducement to pose for pictures would take so much pleasure standing in a small box posing for photos, while pulling silly faces and holding up props? We even booked an ice cream van to arrive for dessert. Adam may have had 99 problems, but not having a 99 wasn't one of them. Hey, I've been pretty restrained with the dad jokes for a while, so give me a break, OK?

Yet all this paled into insignificance when compared with the undisputed highlight of the evening. We hired a mobile video game arcade, housed within a large tent that just about fitted inside our garden. Within were rows of consoles where Adam and his friends were able to play all manner of ultra-violent games. Granted, playing Nintendo and Xbox might not have been the most Jewish *bar mitzvah* ever, unless you're playing *Grand Theft Auto: Golders Green*. Then again, this party cost a 20th of everyone else's *bar mitzvah*, and there's nothing more Jewish than the pleasure of saving money.*

To say our guests enjoyed it would be a massive understatement. This wasn't the usual *bar mitzvah* they were accustomed to. There was no formality, no demands on anyone to behave respectfully, no having to be quiet during speeches and absolutely no pretence about this being a religious rite of passage. Adam's friends from primary school all came: One-Word Freedman, Monotone Williams, Only-Eats-Rice-Cakes Davis and Faraway-Look Daniels. We also had his new friends from secondary

---

* I'm allowed to make that joke, you're not. Unless you're also Jewish, in which case please ignore this footnote and feel free to make these kinds of jokes to your heart's content.

school: Robot-Boy Stephens, Rigidity Rosenberg, No-Eye-Contact Newman and Odd-as-Fuck Levy. Regrettably, some enjoyed it a little too much. The following day we received several complaints from mums and dads – interestingly, all parents of *Coldplays* that Adam had mysteriously befriended – who were livid that their sons were now demanding their *bar mitzvah* party be as cool as this one. A few also complained about their children having been exposed to such inappropriate games, and I spent several days dealing with the fall-out from what became known as 'GTAgate'. But would I change a thing? Definitely not.

At the end of the evening, as Gemma and I were clearing away pizza boxes and trying to calm Edward down because one LEGO lightsaber had allegedly gone astray, Adam wandered into the kitchen.

'That was totally the best *bar mitzvah* ever.'

Wow, now that was rare praise. One boy in Adam's class had a lavish *bar mitzvah* with the theme 'Our Family United by Love'. We accepted that would never be us, so our theme was more 'Our Family United by Junk Food'. And honestly, it was amazing. We didn't dwell on what our son couldn't do but celebrated what he could. And if what he could do was encourage numerous *Coldplays* to overdose on pizza, candyfloss and ice cream while shooting people on some incredibly unsuitable video games, then that was fine by me.

If you've got a family occasion coming up, many congratulations! Or to stick with the theme of this chapter, *mazal tov*! To be clear, the story of Adam's 'un-*bar mitzvah*' is not intended as the definitive how-to guide for making a celebration involving your *Zappa*. This is

simply what worked for us. I still don't know if we made the right decision, or whether we should have pushed Adam to do more, or maybe even allowed him to do less.*
There are many ways to approach occasions like this, and no doubt your celebrations will be just as varied as your children. But before we move on, here are a few pointers.

1. Commit yourself to acceptance

I know accepting your child the way they are is never an easy route. It's no more a magic bullet for parenting than the naughty step or sticker charts. But when you're the parent to a *Zappa*, it's the most powerful tool you have. Be realistic about what they can and can't do, even if it doesn't chime with your pre-existing plans and fantasies.

2. Don't compare your family with other people

This is so much easier said than done. Adam was a summer baby, so we had almost an entire academic year of seeing his peers perform their *bar mitzvahs* with aplomb, followed by extravagant parties. By July the pressure was huge. The best thing we ever did was say 'Fuck

---

* Not sure how that would have been possible. To have made it any less Jewish he'd have needed to cover the pizzas with ham and regrow his foreskin.

it' and move on. So what if their sons gave beautiful speeches and recited numerous prayers in Hebrew? We had pizza and video games!!

3. There are no rules

When planning a family celebration, ban the following words:

Should
Ought
Must
Usually
Expected
Normal

The only thing that matters is making your *Zappa* feel comfortable, and how that is achieved is entirely up to you.

4. Every child is different

A few years later it was time for Zoe's *bat mitzvah*. She wasn't mentally capable of doing anything in synagogue, but we knew she would get a lot from marking this milestone. So, we arranged a celebration at her school and then a second one at her Sunday club. Meanwhile, Dylan wanted to match Adam's complete avoidance of religious observance, but perhaps influenced by his school friends, asked us to spend as much money as possible on one of those over-the-top dinner dances. This would never have been Gemma's or my cup of tea, so I'm not sure how we'd have got out of this while retaining our whole 'It's up to the child' mantra. Just thank God for the COVID pandemic, because his *bar mitzvah* fell during lockdown, hence we managed to escape it altogether.

5. Don't ever consider converting to Judaism

You may be grappling with arranging big birthday parties, confirmations, proms, sweet 16s, or *quinceañeras*, and if they involve trying to accommodate a *Zappa* then they're not going to be easy. Just be grateful that you're not Jewish, because the *bar* and *bat mitzvah* are a real pain, and probably enough to stop you thinking of conversion. Chicken soup and smoked salmon bagels are nice, but you can have them without joining the club.

6. Enjoy it

There are enough sad and shitty moments in life, so try not to turn what should be a rare happy occasion into anything other than joyful. Just do it on yours and your child's terms, and all will be well. Congratulations. *Mazal tov.* ¡*Felicitaciones!*

21

K IS FOR KIDS HAVE THEIR SAY

ADAM: We can say whatever we want?! A whole chapter, just us talking, and you'll record it and write it down? Like, anything we say at all?!

OLLIE: Nah, don't believe it. He'll edit it to make him sound good and make us look like idiots. That's what he normally does.

ADAM: Well, let's see. Fuck. You writing that down? Fuck. Shit. Cunt. Erm …

DYLAN: Wank.

ADAM: Shut up, Dylan.

OLLIE: He doesn't care about swearing, Dad swears all the time. I bet those words are in the book already. He probably told that story about you saying 'Fuck' when you read it on a T-shirt.

ADAM: Oh, he always goes on about that and it's probably not even true.

OLLIE: Yeah, 'cos you still can't read.

DYLAN: Yeah, you still can't read.

OLLIE: Shut up, Dylan.

BAILEY: Can I have a drink?

ADAM: So, what do we talk about?

OLLIE: How Dad's written a book about his children even though he spends half the year 'on tour'.

ADAM: Yeah, 'on tour'.

DYLAN: Haha. 'On tour'.

ADAM: Shut up, Dylan.

EDWARD: There's a new *Star Wars* LEGO set I want. Can I have the next two years of pocket money in advance?

OLLIE: Stop going on about LEGO and let me and Adam do the talking.

ADAM: Zoe, what are you doing?

ZOE: Nuffing.

BAILEY: Can I have a drink?

OLLIE: Daddy will get it after we've done this.

ADAM: OK, so what shall we say?

OLLIE: Just agree with everything in the book.

ADAM: But I've not read it.

DYLAN: 'Cos you can't read.

ADAM: Shut up, Dylan.

DYLAN: I know you really love me, Adam.

OLLIE: You don't need to read it. I can tell you everything in it. I supposedly don't use deodorant. Edward goes on and on about LEGO.

EDWARD: LEGO, LEGO, LEGO, LEGO.

OLLIE: Zoe is amazing 'cos he loves her more than the rest of us.

ADAM: He only adopted her for Facebook likes. What you doing, Zoe?

ZOE: Nuffing.

OLLIE: You're always swearing and were crap at school. Bailey won't ever shut up. And Dylan is always talking shit about stuff he's seen on YouTube.

DYLAN: Well, that's kinda true.

ADAM: Shut up, Dylan.

OLLIE: And that's probably it, padded out for four hundred pages, all to make him look good. And I bet he mentions 'Pubesgate' just to embarrass me.

ADAM: What idiots are going to want to read that?

BAILEY: Can I have a drink?

22

V IS FOR VARIOUS TIMES MY CHILDREN HAVE HUMILIATED ME

A few years ago I saw a movie called Us. If you've not seen it, skip the following sentences as they contain spoilers. It's a psychological horror film written and directed by Jordan Peele, based on the idea that somewhere underground there are evil doppelgängers of everyone in the world. They're barely verbal and appear to be entirely malevolent. It's meant to be a scary idea, but as I watched it an even more terrible thought occurred to me: maybe we're the bad Blakers and somewhere there's a nice version of our family. Perhaps the real me even has a full head of hair, and doesn't have chronic athlete's foot and piles.

I covered my children's dubious social skills in Chapter 2, but I'd hate you to think that was a true reflection of what my kids are like. Believe me, they're much worse. To that end, allow me to share some of the other occasions Gemma and I have suffered humiliation at the hands of our children. In no particular order, let's begin with:

1. 'Policegate'

Once, while driving down the A5, I was pulled over by the police. As the officer approached my car, what I needed was for the children in the back to be quiet. What I got was something else entirely.

'Yes!!' screeched Dylan, high-fiving Edward. 'Dad's going to prison! No homework tonight!'

Adam had more important issues on his mind. 'Dad, if you go to prison, do you think you'll be someone's punk, or will you be the daddy?'

The policeman started speaking to me through my wound-down window, but I couldn't hear a word for all the chaos in the car, nor could he concentrate on whatever he wanted to say because the kids had now ceased asking me their ridiculous questions and turned their attention to him.

'Hey, cop', said Adam. 'Have you got a taser?' Everyone started squealing in excitement.

Then Dylan had a brainwave. 'Hey, Adam, get out your phone and film this. We can put it on YouTube and we'll all be famous!'

He and Adam started making these hashtag signs with their fingers, which one of their idiot friends must have told them is super-cool. Sorry, super-sick.

'Nice kids you've got,' the police officer remarked, kindly ignoring the phone camera now being held inches from his face.

From here, things actually got worse, as Edward attempted to use a Jedi mind trick to convince the policeman 'we're not the Jews you're looking for'. It turned out it was merely that one of my brake lights had gone, but the officer was so shocked by his brief encounter with my boys that it looked like he'd have rather volunteered for a stint with the riot squad. At least the Extinction Rebellion protesters don't also go on and on about *Star Wars*. Or dinosaurs. Or Marvel movies. Or LEGO.

The police officer quickly made his way back to his car, while I called out after him. 'Arrest me!' I yelled. 'I could do with a quiet night in the cells.'

2. 'Passovergate'

Oy, Passover. If you didn't know, Passover is an annual Jewish holiday which celebrates the time that the children of Israel escaped from being slaves in Egypt. You may have read the story in the early part of the Bible; in fairness, by the standards of the rest of the Old Testament, it's one of the more dramatic and interesting bits. The festival lasts eight days, during which time Jews are meant to avoid bread and all other leavened products. Instead, we eat these crackers called *matzah*, which taste like cardboard and give you either horrific constipation or terrible diarrhoea.* What a way to celebrate our freedom from slavery!

The centrepiece of Passover is the family meal on the first night, known as the *seder*. Depending on whose *seder* you go to, this is either a very dull religious service

---

* Time doesn't permit me to elaborate on how eating *matzah* can cause two seemingly contradictory effects. You'll just have to trust me when I say eating it will fuck with your stomach, one way or another.

that will last for hours, or a glorified dinner party, although both cases will probably involve Jews doing what they do best, which is arguing with each other. There's a depiction of a particularly dreadful one in an episode of *Curb Your Enthusiasm*, to which Larry David invites a sex offender. I imagine when they were developing this storyline, the writers' room envisaged that Larry welcoming a paedophile would be the ultimate in terrible *seders*. Those writers had never been to a Blaker family *seder*.

The worst – and trust me, there's some competition – was the year Gemma invited local friends to join us. What was she thinking? Why would she want an audience for the mortification that was to come? Not only that, but she had invited the best-behaved family we knew, the ultimate *Coldplays*, who would inevitably be horrified by the experience.

I won't name the family in question, but I don't need to because we never referred to them by their real surname anyway. We always knew them as the Flanders, named after the next-door neighbours in *The Simpsons*. Yes, I'm aware that makes me Homer but, hey, if the cap fits. The similarity was just too striking: both Flanders families are religious, good-natured, cheery and seemingly perfect, especially when viewed in contrast with their neighbours. The only major difference is that rather than having two angelic boys – Rod and Todd – these Flanders have two girls, who are pretty much the opposite of my famously belligerent Blakers. While my boys will fight each other to the death over a packet of Maltesers, the Flanders girls will happily share a stick of celery. My boys spend the evening killing people on video games and hurling Argos catalogues at my head; the Flanders will play charades and enjoy each other's company. My children aren't satisfied in the holidays unless they've been to a theme park and spent a fortune in the gift shop. I once asked Mr Flanders what they had planned for the summer, and he told me they'd given each of their daughters a British prime minister whose life and career they were to research. The fun never ends in their house!

Given this, you can imagine their reaction when they entered our home for the *seder*. Edward was the first child to come downstairs to greet them, only rather than wearing the smart clothes we'd expected, he appeared in a full LEGO-man costume, complete with an oversized plastic head.

'Why are you wearing that to the *seder*?' I asked.

A muffled voice rose from the yellow depths. 'You told me to put on my best outfit. Adam said this was what I liked the best so I should put it on.'

I don't know how many times I'd told him, if you start any sentence with the words 'Adam said', you need to take ten minutes to reconsider, and then do the opposite.

We eventually started the service, and the Flanders girls had lots of questions to ask, as is traditional at the *seder*.

'Daddy, why did Pharaoh not set the Jews free after the first of the plagues?' Decent question.

'Mummy, why did God make us slaves to begin with?' Can't fault that one either.

Now it was Dylan's turn to ask a question. 'Daddy, why are Quavers never on offer in Tesco?'

'What?!'

'Well, everything seems to be on offer at some point and they've had Wotsits and Hula Hoops half-price, but they never seem to have Quavers. Is this a conspiracy? I was watching a video on YouTube that said if you don't reject cookie settings then the government know what you're looking at and they pass your information to the supermarkets to make sure the things you want aren't on sale. And I've been googling Quavers to see when they might be on sale, and I think that's why they aren't.'

Gemma looked at him bemused. 'Why are you asking this now?'

'You said we had to prepare questions for the *seder*. I have others.' He held up three sheets of A4 covered in mostly illegible scribble. I could just about make out the word 'zombies' many times over.

This was a high point when it came to my children's involvement in the *seder*. I shortly discovered Adam was using a prayer book in which each page had been covered over by articles cut out from *Match of the Day Magazine*. The holy texts were now barely visible as he'd used Pritt Stick to obscure them with features about Cristiano Ronaldo and Lionel Messi.

Then, when invited to sing a Passover song, The Bailey performed a near perfect rendition of 'Away in a Manger'. I pointed out to Mrs Flanders that since the Last Supper was technically a *seder*, The Bailey's mentions of Little Lord Jesus weren't as inappropriate as one might initially think.

The final nail in the coffin was when Zoe wandered off, only to return to the table holding a forbidden slice of bread. Forget Larry David's paedophile friend; Gary Glitter would be more welcome at the *seder* than a piece of Hovis. This was the last straw for the Flanders, and they quickly made their excuses and cut the evening short. We were left to tell the story of the Children of Israel on our own, and to contemplate that if it had been the Children of Blaker instead, then God would probably have chosen to leave them in Egypt.

3. 'Goatgate'

You'd think at this point that nothing would surprise me when it comes to my children. It says a lot about them that they still manage to astonish me on a regular basis. And possibly no incident in recent years has staggered me more than 'Goatgate'.

As I said in the Introduction, Edward is technically a *Coldplay*, and he'll remain this way unless he decides to pursue a diagnosis in later life. Many people with ASD only receive confirmation in adulthood. Perhaps one day this will be Edward, but for now we felt there was no huge benefit to getting him assessed, and I hope he won't feel we made a bad choice. Yet while he may not have a label, Edward can in many ways out-autistic Adam and Dylan combined.

Last November I had a phone call from the head of year at Edward's new secondary school. Having only just started, Edward had already managed to get himself banned from the computer room. As Mrs Wilson explained, he was quite upset about it, so she felt it best to call his parents to fill them in on what had happened. It appeared that since he wasn't very sporty and didn't want to play football at lunchtimes, Edward had been sneaking back inside to use the computers, which were out of bounds apart from during ICT lessons. He was so small that no one had ever seen him wandering the corridors, and even when a teacher entered the computer room they hadn't noticed him slouched in front of a keyboard. Sadly, he'd been caught out because of his internet search history.

This is where the story takes an unusual turn. Given that Edward is 12 years old and about to enter puberty, you might imagine he was searching for hardcore pornography. It would hardly be unusual for a boy his age. I once found Adam trying to see if you can get Pornhub on a TomTom.* But I'd hope by now you know lovely, sweet Edward well enough to guess he wasn't looking for anything like that. You're probably imagining he was googling dinosaurs, LEGO, or *Star Wars*. Maybe Marvel movies. But no, it was none of these. His search term was consistently 'Brilliant goats'.

Mrs Wilson was as surprised as anyone. She asked Edward why he was creeping into the computer room to google 'Brilliant goats'.

'I like looking at photos of goats,' he replied nonchalantly.

'Oh, you mean G.O.A.T., as in greatest of all time?'

'No, the animal goat.'

Mrs Wilson was still confused. 'OK, Edward, but why "brilliant goats" instead of just "goats"?'

Edward was equally baffled by what to him was such

---

* FYI you can't, although terms like 'right there' and 'turn around when possible' can sound sexy depending on which voice you opt for.

a stupid question. 'I don't like looking at any old goats. I only want to look at the brilliant ones.' Fair enough. Who'd want to look at a shit goat?

We'd known about Edward's love of goats since he did a presentation regarding them at the end of Year Six. Yet even I was taken aback by the apparent depth of his passion. I just hope he grows out of searching for photos of cute kids, because one day that really will be seriously inappropriate.

4. 'Toiletgate'

About three years ago we were having some work done in the house. If you visited today, you wouldn't believe this because the way the children have systematically destroyed our home means it feels more 1820s than 2020s. I think the distressed look is in vogue, so perhaps I should grateful.

One of the jobs our builders were undertaking was updating Gemma's and my ensuite bathroom. I'm aware it sounds rather grand having an ensuite to ourselves, but even the world's biggest sadomasochist would balk at using our family bathroom. I know it can take many years for little boys, even *Coldplays*, to learn how to wee straight but mine … well, I was going to say take the piss, but if only they did. Rather than take it, they leave it; not just unflushed in the bowl, but on the seat, in puddles on the floor, dribbling down the walls and in places physics would suggest simply couldn't be performed by a child standing in front of the toilet. Conspiracy theorists would have a field day and no doubt suggest the presence of a second shooter hidden behind the bathtub. If my boys ever decide to attend Glastonbury, they'll think the facilities are positively palatial.

This wasn't a quick job, and while the builders tried their best to limit the disruption – I pleaded with them, 'Please don't make me use the kids' bathroom. I'll pay you anything you want!!' – there was one evening when our new toilet was out of action. They had fixed the porcelain in place, grouted around it but not finished the plumbing, so it wasn't to be used since it couldn't be flushed. The builders left for the day, and we gathered the children for a family meeting.

'Please can everyone make sure they don't use our bathroom.' Everyone nodded while barely taking their eyes off the screens they were holding. I was confident the message had been received and understood.

Famous last words. Barely half an hour later, Gemma and I were talking in the kitchen when I felt a drop of water on my head. Strange, I thought. Where's that coming from? I looked up to see water dripping through the ceiling. I say dripping, but it soon became pouring and, very quickly after that, torrential. Within a couple of minutes, there was an enormous hole where the ceiling used to be, through which water was cascading like Niagara Falls.

One of the children – let's leave them nameless – had forgotten my instruction from less than 30 minutes earlier, and decided to use our bathroom. In the culprit's defence, the family bathroom had been occupied, but the downstairs toilet was available, so why they trotted off to our room is anyone's guess. I wouldn't mind, but they never normally flush the toilet! Had the perpetrator just done a pee and left it, for once this would have been a good thing. Instead, they broke the habit of a lifetime, flushed it away, and immediately gave our kitchen a black hole bigger than the one in Calcutta.

It was a chastening experience when, the next morning, the builders arrived and saw the dark void in the ceiling.* Being completely useless at anything practical, I've always found interactions with builders intimidating. Likewise mechanics, plumbers, electricians and the like. But this was a whole different level.

'I thought I told you not to use that toilet, mate. Did you not tell the kids?'

It's one thing feeling inadequate because you don't know what an RSJ is. That I can cope with; they probably wouldn't be able to explain the comedy rule of three to me. But I've never felt like such a shit parent. I actually lied and said it was me who forgot. It seemed preferable to take the rap myself, rather than admit my words of warning had been completely ignored by the children.

The humiliation didn't end there. We were now left with a black hole the enormity of which would have interested Stephen Hawking, and as anyone who's had to make a claim on their building insurance will know, it's never swift. First an assessor came to inspect the damage, then sometime later two approved builders arrived and each prepared a quote. It took weeks, during which any visitor to our house would have judged us for living in such squalor or, if they heard the reason, for doing such a bad job at parenting. I've never been so grateful for having no friends coming into our home.

---

* Don't believe me? See the photos.

Of course, very occasionally we do have guests round, and I wish I could tell you they were good experiences. Alas, let me conclude this chapter with yet another anecdote from *The Blaker Book of Misery* ...

5. 'Nipkinsgate'

Oh God, I cringe just thinking about this. So, as you should realise by now, no one in my house can get along. If it's not the children taking every word said to them utterly literally – let's not revisit 'Batsignalgate' – it's the incessant name-calling. Some of it is harmless, and I can just about tolerate Adam calling me a 'wanger'. Trust me, I've been called worse on Twitter. But I'm an adult and have fairly thick skin.* The kids, on the other hand, aren't as mature, nor are they professional comics who've been toughened up by performing for difficult audiences. And if Dylan's memes are anything to go by, he probably never will be a comedian either. That's possibly for the best because he, more than any of the others, gets very distressed when it comes to insults, especially those from his siblings.

Of all the names he's been called, the most upsetting to him was 'Nipkins'. I can't truthfully explain why Adam and Ollie started using this or where it came from. I do remember that it was originally 'Granny Nipkins' and that it then got shortened to just 'Nipkins', but I've no idea where they'd heard it. I'm tempted to say a book or TV show, and given their lack of interest in reading, it

---

* Please don't take this as an invitation to test just how thick my skin is.

must have been the latter. The crucial point is that they started calling him 'Nipkins' and Dylan absolutely hated it. Which, as you should have guessed, meant Adam and Ollie did it even more.

'Shut up, Nipkins!'

'What are you watching, Nipkins?'

'Lend us your charger cable, Nipkins!'

Any of these would have caused Dylan to burst into tears and make me or Gemma interrupt whatever we were doing. In her case, cooking or working; in mine, more likely watching football. At least I'm honest! Dylan hated this name so much, even one of us telling the older boys to stop calling him 'Nipkins' could itself provoke crying. Dylan was so distraught that we had to arrange a family meeting in which we announced a total ban of what Gemma tactfully called the 'N-word'.

All was fine, and Adam and Ollie adhered to the prohibition. However, a few weeks later we had a good friend round for lunch. She was bringing her new boyfriend, David, to meet us and he just so happened to be Afro-Caribbean. Our old social worker from Hackney would have been very impressed. Well, that is until the boys started arguing over some chocolates that David had brought for dessert.

'I'm having first!' demanded Dylan.

'Shut up, idiot,' replied Ollie.

Dylan, always easy to upset, cried out in the direction of the kitchen. 'Mum!! Ollie called me an idiot!!'

At this point, probably worrying that his gift had inadvertently caused an argument between our boys, David tried to get involved. 'Come on, everyone's going to get a chocolate. You don't need to call him an idiot.'

'Oh, it's fine. We can call him that. Mummy and Daddy just said we shouldn't use the N-word.'

I am not sure David could believe what he'd heard. 'The N-word?'

Before I could explain, Ollie answered, 'Yes, we used to say it all the time, but we've been told we can't say it now.'

Unsurprisingly, David looked horrified. I jumped in to explain this meant 'Nipkins', although I am not entirely sure David was convinced by this rather fanciful-sounding story. And so our attempts to mollify Dylan and bring peace to the house had unintentionally made us look like the world's most racist family. We aren't, but to avoid all doubt I now insist that this toe-curlingly embarrassing incident be referred to by its full name – 'Nipkinsgate' – rather than the more misleading 'N-wordgate'.

23

R IS FOR ROUTINES

Whether you have one *Zappa*; one *Zappa* plus one or more *Coldplays*; or three *Zappas* and three who-knows-what-they-are – and if that's you, I'm afraid you're infringing my copyright and will be hearing from my lawyer – it's important to put routines in place. Morning routine, leaving for school routine, bathtime routine, bedtime routine, tearing your hair out because no one will go to sleep routine.*

All children can be challenging at these moments, and *Zappas* even more so. The good news is that many children with special needs, especially those with ASD, will appreciate a clear routine, whether they'd willingly admit it or not. There may be resistance at first, but children with autism tend to like repetition and sameness, so routines will come naturally and ultimately bring comfort. The bad news is that it might not be as easy as it sounds, at least if our experiences are anything to go by, because our attempts to implement routines have

---

* I'd love to think this is the reason for my receding hairline and that when the kids mature it will all grow back.

not been an unqualified success. In fact, the best advice I can give in this chapter is to see what our house looks like in the morning and try to achieve the exact opposite.

Part of this may be a function of having too many children; part of it may be that raising three *Zappas* is asking too much of anyone; and part of it is probably good old Blaker belligerence. I can't say for sure, but I do know that, despite our best efforts, getting everyone ready for school is never as simple as I think it should be. I'll admit, this has led to resentment on my part. I want things to be stress-free in the morning, and the fact that they never are has caused no little bitterness. Not to my children, I should add. No, my malice is aimed entirely at Michael McIntyre.

Before I'm accused of being a typically sour comedian, unable to accept other performers' achievements, let me explain. This is nothing to do with Michael McIntyre being ever so slightly more successful than me. It's simply because Michael McIntyre performs routines about how hard it is parenting two children. Michael, you've got literally a third of our children!* And not only that. To the best of my knowledge Michael has two *Coldplays*. I can't be the only one watching him perform stand-up about his boys' night-time routine who's thinking this is a breeze. Frankly, going on national TV and moaning about anything so easy is taking ... well, taking the Michael.

What is probably his most famous skit on this topic has had over 2.4 million views on YouTube and is listed

---

* Well, not literally, obviously, because that would imply two of our children are also his, which would be good because he could afford to buy them as many chargers as they needed.

under the title 'People Without Children Have NO IDEA What It's Like!' No, Michael, those of you with two *Coldplays* have no idea what it's like. The routine goes something like this.

> If you've got children, leaving the house takes forever because it's all 'Come downstairs, Lucas! Where are your shoes? Go find your shoes. When did you last have your shoes? Stand still while I do up your zip. If you don't come downstairs, Oscar, we're leaving without you.

And that's it! It took him less than three minutes. With all due respect, Michael, if these two children are giving you that much difficulty, you wouldn't want to spend any time in my house because you'd have a coronary. *This* is what our morning routine is like.

7.29 a.m.

It's half an hour before we leave for school and although the house is quiet, Gemma and I have been up for some time, steeling ourselves for what's to come. *Operation: Get Everyone to School* isn't simple, but at least everything feasible has been done in advance to make the process as painless as possible. Bags by the door arranged in age order. Breakfast on the table organised by the children's ever-changing taste and sound preferences. Medications laid out neatly by each child's preferred swallowing method. Shoes by the stairs, waiting for feet. Some of us are prepared, Michael.

7.30 a.m.

Reluctantly, bodies emerge from bedrooms and, as the noise and fighting begin, the calm of the morning is shattered.

'Everyone, can you please come downstairs!! Bailey, have you brushed your teeth?'

Even though she's the youngest, she wants to be independent and do everything herself. However, it's all done at a pace somewhere between ponderous and glacial, and she unhelpfully answers every question regarding her progress, 'Noyes' or 'Yesno'.

'████, █████, █████, ██████, have you brushed your teeth?'

The names have been redacted to spare the embarrassment of the four children to whom I need to ask this question. I would hate to humiliate these boys by suggesting that even at their age they need reminding to perform basic oral hygiene.

7.35 a.m.

Having helped Zoe brush her teeth – the one teenager for whom this feels reasonable – I start the long job of readying her for school, because she can't get dressed independently, let alone sort out her glasses and hearing aid. It feels cruel to put on the latter before she leaves the house, since at this point the noise is so horrific, deafness would be a blessing.

I must admit partial responsibility for the noise, because this isn't a time for rational debate. School mornings are when I turn into a drill sergeant and will shout at anyone and everyone I feel needs geeing up. Which, let's face it, means everyone. This even includes Zoe, as in the mornings she can be at her most pugnacious, especially when time is of the essence. Never mind that her bus will be arriving in five minutes. If she wants to play with her dolly or is trying to expand her linguistic expertise by watching *Peppa Pig* in Punjabi, there's nothing in the world that's going to persuade her otherwise. Yes, I know, no one asked us to adopt her.

7.39 a.m.

The noise in the house is about to get a whole lot louder because Ollie is stomping downstairs in an absolute fury, shouting at Gemma.

'Where's my protractor?! I need my protractor and I'm going to get a detention and it's all your fault! What have you done with it, woman?! If you'd just stop reading your stupid books and cooking your disgusting food, maybe you'd have time to be a proper mother and find my protractor!!'

Let's briefly overlook the worrying anger issues and reprehensible rudeness to his mother. Instead, let's turn our attention to the bizarre idea that Gemma is responsible for losing Ollie's protractor. It would be a strange notion just once, but to compound the improbability, these accusations are made every single day. It's as though he genuinely imagines Gemma waits until he's asleep, then creeps into his room and steals his protractor for her own gratification. Maybe he thinks that as soon as he's gone to school, she spends the rest of the day going around the house measuring angles. God knows where his protractors do end up, but we've needed to replace so much lost stationery over the past few years I think we're personally keeping WHSmith in business. We find the best approach in these moments is to remain silent. Don't engage, it won't get you anywhere. Anyway, I'm too busy trying to get Zoe's shoes on, while she watches what I've discovered is called ਪੱਪਾ ਪਿਗ.

7.42 a.m.

Having failed to mollify him, Ollie is now hurling cushions off the sofa, half looking for his protractor, half in a Hulk-like rage. 'Mr McGee, don't make Ollie angry. You wouldn't like him when he's angry.' However, as a result of his assault on our furniture, he inadvertently uncovers an enormous pile of jellybeans, which prompts every member of the family to stop what they're doing and gather around the newly discovered sweets. Even Edward, who normally wouldn't stop playing with his LEGO if our house were engulfed by an inferno.

A little backstory. Three years ago, a visitor to the house brought a big box of Jelly Belly gourmet jellybeans that simply vanished. We hunted everywhere; inquests were held; fingers of blame were pointed at the likely culprits. Yet no amount of investigation got us anywhere. Had our guest brought round a tray of dried fruit no one would have cared, but these jellybeans had brought every child downstairs to bagsy their favourite flavours. We'd already had threats of violence over the Very Cherry beans, universally beloved in our house, yet also slightly feared for their resemblance to Cinnamon.* Then the box disappeared, and the jellybeans became something of a legend in our house – a confectionery *Mary Celeste* – mentioned every couple of months, when new theories would be posited.

Fast forward three years and, having blamed Adam and Ollie for the past 36 months, it turns out the jellybeans had simply fallen between the sofa cushions, which given the endless school meetings and hospital appointments we'd never had time to clean. It's no surprise then that everyone is now gathered round in awe. Edward is boldly claiming, 'This is the greatest day in my entire life!'† Meanwhile, Dylan is counting the beans to ascertain if any had been eaten before their disappearance. I'd be thrilled if one day Dylan did graduate to become a figurative bean counter, but at this point I must make do with being father to a literal bean counter.

Ordinarily, I'd have been delighted we'd finally resolved the mystery of 'Jellybeangate', but not 18 minutes before leaving for school. Sadly, because of this discovery, no one is putting on their shoes or coats and they've all quickly descended into fighting over who

---

* No one wants the horrible taste of cinnamon in their mouth, let alone those with sensory issues. Quite why Jelly Belly make the nicest and the most disgusting of their flavours look so similar is beyond me. I can only put it down to someone at the company being a sadistic bastard.

† Previous holders of this title have included the day his LEGO Death Star arrived, the launch day of Season 2 of *The Mandalorian* and the day he was allowed into the computer room at school to search for brilliant goats.

should get to eat the fluff-encrusted jellybeans. Forget the school run; there's never an ideal time to find yourself refereeing a full-on death-match between an autistic teenager and a sugar-crazed eight-year-old.

7.45 a.m.

Having negotiated a truce and divided up the jellybeans equally – albeit with Adam and Ollie getting double after they demanded reparations for being falsely accused of jellybean embezzlement – I'm back trying to put shoes on Zoe. It's now even harder to get her dressed since she's unable to help, being too busy eating her antique sweets. This is fine, however, since – momentarily – everyone is happy. Not least Gemma, who's basking in the joy of an unexpected meal she didn't have to wash up. The cereals and bowls have already been put away, while the children enjoy a nutritious breakfast of stale, dusty jellybeans. Part of their five-a-day; sugary treats, that is.

7.47 a.m.

I'm still dressing Zoe when Dylan ambles over with an urgent question. I wonder if by this point you've got to know him sufficiently well to guess which of the following it is:

A. 'Can I have some money for after school?'
B. 'Can you pick me up from a friend's house?'
C. 'What's for dinner tonight?'
D. 'Daddy, if you could choose to be a pig or a wolf, what would you be?'

If you answered A, B or C, then either you haven't been paying attention or I've done a really crap job at describing my third son. Hopefully, you'll have guessed correctly and will appreciate by now that this kind of question is completely normal for him, even amid the morning chaos. The only good news is that these dilemmas don't usually require an answer since this isn't really a conversation, it's just a stream of consciousness.

'I would be a wolf, no a pig, no a wolf, no a pig, no an eagle. Actually, I was thinking last night that pigs and wolves are virtually the same thing except wolves are hairy.'

I should probably correct his misunderstanding of the animal kingdom, but I'm still busy with Zoe, who, while putting on her shoes, has removed her hearing aid seven times.

7.49 a.m.

I finally have Zoe dressed – but who am I kidding?! We both know that her hearing aid will come off another dozen times before the bus comes – when I notice that Adam is leaving for college, in the bleak midwinter, wearing the same shorts and T-shirt he just slept in. Like a total idiot, I make the mistake of pointing this out. He briefly stops rifling through my wallet to shout, 'Stop micro-managing me! Sort your own life out before you get involved with mine!' At least pickpockets in the street just take your cash. They don't feel the need to verbally abuse and parent shame you while they're at it.

7.51 a.m.

The Bailey has finished eating her jellybeans but has decided she now wants to put on make-up. This despite the fact Gemma almost never wears make-up, so she's obviously learnt this from a YouTube channel we're too overwhelmed to stop her watching. Also, despite the fact her school obviously doesn't allow an eight-year-old to wear make-up, because it's a primary school, not *Minipops* or Kim Kardashian's Instagram.*

Of course, anyone that knows The Bailey will be aware that merely explaining that her school forbids make-up isn't going to wash (the make-up off her face). Remember, she's a Blaker and so she thinks the normal rules don't apply to her. Hence, another crucial couple of minutes are lost as I try to explain that in fact the normal rules *do* apply to her, and that just because Niki and Gabi are wearing this shade of eye shadow doesn't mean she should too. Especially not to school. Especially seeing that she's eight years old.

7.53 a.m.

The Bailey has taken off her make-up – using the remover recommended by Zoella, obvs, girlfriend – and with seven minutes left until it's time to leave the house, we're roughly back on track. Zoe has taken her hearing

---

* By a funny coincidence, there's a Jewish primary school in London called North West. However, I believe it's named after its location rather than the make-up wearing nine-year-old daughter of Kim Kardashian, who's probably one of The Bailey's online role models.

aid off another six times, and I've now given up and decided to keep it in my pocket until her bus arrives. Why didn't I think of that earlier? More worryingly, she has managed to lose her glasses and I've enlisted everyone else to join the hunt, with the promise of £1 for the person that finds them. You didn't think they'd help me for nothing, did you? Everyone joins in, even Ollie, who had long since abandoned the search for the protractor in favour of eating his double-share of the primaeval jellybeans. Everyone except one child, that is, who wishes to ask another question. I wonder if by this point you've got to know my children sufficiently well to guess which of them it is.

A. Adam
B. The Bailey
C. Edward
D. Dylan

Again, if you answered A, B or C, then either you haven't been paying attention or I've done a really crap job at describing my third son. And what a question it is.

'Daddy, why did our Lord Jesus Christ die for our sins on the cross?'

This time I feel compelled to postpone the search for Zoe's glasses in order to reply. 'Dylan, we're Jewish.'

There's a stunned silence, as though Dylan has never heard this before. Even more remarkable given he's attended a Jewish school every day for the past ten years.

'So, you're saying you don't care about Jesus? I thought you said we should care about every living thing, so why doesn't Jesus count?'

At this point, I make a mental note to email the speech therapist who taught this child to speak and demand an apology.

7.55 a.m.

Adam finds the glasses thrown behind the sofa and immediately demands his pound. Which is fine, I did offer it, but he's just stolen £20, so asking for an extra 5 per cent feels cheeky, even by Adam's standards. I can't moan, because losing Zoe's glasses would be even worse, so I pay up and Adam leaves for college, still in his shorts and T-shirt. I try to give him a hug, but he screams, 'Ugh, you're squashing my vagina!' Obviously, I let go of him because what boy can learn successfully, even his Level 1 college course, with a squashed vagina? Clearly his course isn't Introduction to Human Biology.

7.56 a.m.

Remarkably, Zoe's bus arrives. It appears that the driver's alarm has worked and he's woken on time; the escort hasn't needed an emergency hernia operation; there's no rain or snow; the tyres are inflated; the wiper blades haven't cracked; none of the kids on the bus have needed a change of clothing; and there isn't a partial eclipse of the moon. Luckily, I remember that Zoe's hearing aid is in my pocket and I pop it on her head, knowing that if she takes it off now, it's Helen's problem. Of course, that's nonsense. If she loses it on the bus, as has happened several times, it's Muggins Blaker who will end up dealing with the hospital to get a replacement. Remember that suggestion to befriend the consultant's secretary and learn their direct number? *This* is when you need it.

7.58 a.m.

With Zoe safely on her transport, we've a fighting chance of not being stuck in traffic. Adam has taken himself and his vagina to the bus stop; Ollie has headed off to school, either with or without a protractor, which I'm sure he's never used anyway, and he actually meant calculator; and Dylan and The Bailey are strapped in the car, and finally I'm pulling off the drive. And breathe ...

8.03 a.m.

I'm already stuck in stand-still traffic on the Edgware Road, when I realise I've accidentally left Edward at home and have to go back to get him. Oh, and Michael, if by some small chance you're reading this and still think your morning routine is hard, I was playing mine down because I'd be too embarrassed for readers to find out how chaotic our house really is.

Given the turmoil I've just described, you may not want my advice, but I'll offer it regardless.

1. *Zappas* need and usually want a strict routine

For many children with SEN, especially those with ASD, routines can be a great tool that will help them cope with possibly anxiety-inducing situations.

2. Display their routine somewhere visible

A visual tool such as a poster on the wall or fridge door will help your child understand their routine. If they find reading difficult, you could make it entirely graphic – a bowl to symbolise breakfast, a tube of toothpaste to represent brushing their teeth, a packet of Jelly Belly to denote stopping for ten minutes to argue about sweets they've discovered under the sofa.

3. Employ positive reinforcement

Your *Zappa* could be encouraged with motivation such as a sticker chart to reward completion of tasks. Getting dressed quickly: one gold star. Brushing your teeth: two gold stars. Not asking any ridiculous questions about whether their father would rather be a dolphin or a sheep because you watched a video on YouTube about how sheep are actually alien life-forms who one day will take over the planet: 20 gold stars.

4. Don't try to do too much at once

Rome wasn't built in a day, so get your child into a consistent schedule, then gradually add new tasks into the routine. Make sure to tackle essentials like getting dressed and combing their hair, before moving on to the really challenging stuff like refraining from rifling through your wallet in search of bank notes.

5. Read this chapter again

The best advice I can give is simply to try to impose a routine better than we have. So re-read this chapter and learn from my mistakes, because despite all my endeavours it never quite goes to plan.

I should be grateful we're able to have a going to school routine again, because there was a horrible period when we dreamed of once more suffering this anarchy in the morning. Which brings me to ...

24

H IS FOR HOME SCHOOL

This chapter is all about our experiences during the COVID-19 pandemic. Remember that? It might have passed you by. And if you're reading this in the 22nd century, this section might explain why your grandparents couldn't add up and wouldn't have known an oxbow lake if it hit them in the face.

The pandemic was a hard time for everyone: NHS staff, shop owners, anyone with no interest in starting a podcast. From my perspective, I can tell you that at a time of enforced lockdown having six children suddenly seemed like it was a bad idea. Because whereas many people complained that their time in quarantine was painfully quiet with no company, mine was an all-day cacophony of noise. I couldn't work without someone interrupting me with:

'Dylan's annoying me!'

'What time is supper?'

'Zoe's annoying me!'

'I can't find my shoes.'

'Adam's annoying me!'

'Can I have a drink?'

'Tell Edward it's my turn on the Xbox.'

'The internet's not working!'

'Tell Dylan it's my turn on the Xbox.'

'Transfer me £10.'

'Dylan and Edward have broken the Xbox.'

Considering several of these children have sensory issues around noise, they can't half produce a racket. Social distancing was also hard as a large family. Every time we went out for one of our daily walks I had angry reactions from people who thought I was running an illicit school trip. Even worse, with eight of us stuck in the house together, we permanently had an illegal social gathering.* I did briefly consider furloughing Adam and Ollie until the end of this period. Let Rishi Sunak pay 80 per cent of their pocket money, and then hopefully welcome them back to the family at a later date. They wouldn't have been allowed do any chores, but since they weren't doing them anyway that would hardly have been a great loss.

As tempting as it was, we soldiered on and addressed the real nightmare, which was home school.† By all accounts, this was a hard enough challenge for parents of *Coldplays*, but for those of us with *Zappas* in the house it was a near impossible job. Some of our kids might not be made for school, but that doesn't take away from the

---

* Boris Johnson had 'Partygate' and for Keir Starmer it was 'Beergate' (aka 'Currygate'), but they had nothing on 'Blakergate'.

† It's sometimes written all one word as 'homeschool', but after abbreviating SEN, I feel I'm owed this small boost towards reaching my word count.

fact they need the routine it provides. Without it, they can become bored and possibly destructive. Zoe especially requires the regimen of school as she needs to be constantly occupied. She might happily sit on the sofa watching her iPad for a while, but after an hour is liable to wander off to perform acts of minor vandalism. Fair enough, *Peppa Pig* in Gujarati doesn't look all it's cracked up to be.

Even Adam and Dylan, as much as they'd claim not to like school, are much the better for it. This is why the school holidays are so challenging. Without the structure of lessons, they'll float around the house starting arguments with anyone with whom they come into contact. I used to think Adam had a special knack for this, but Dylan is very much the new and improved model. He's an iPhone 14 Pro to Adam's iPhone XS. Our younger children can be sitting quietly at the weekend – Edward playing with his LEGO, The Bailey watching an age-inappropriate video and Zoe tearing down strips of wallpaper – and within 30 seconds of Dylan coming downstairs, everyone will be at each other's throats and at least two members of the family will be crying. One of them usually being me.

Let's also remember, many *Zappas* have EHCPs that include a considerable amount of LSA time. Consequently, they're used to someone supporting them through large parts of the day. Adam became very reliant on his LSA in primary school, who was in equal measure his support assistant, minder, handler, translator and slave. I always imagined him spending lessons eating grapes on a wicker throne while Miss Hill did his work for him. Certainly, the artwork he brought home was always of a suspiciously high standard, that is until Miss Hill was replaced with Mrs Forest, since the latter was apparently shit at drawing. So, while parents of *Coldplays* had to take on the difficult job of replacing their kids' teachers, we were doing this and trying to substitute for their LSAs too.

In fairness to the government – not a statement one makes too often regarding the pandemic – there was recognition of the extra challenge facing parents of *Zappas*. Schools were forced to close during lockdown, but there were provisions to support 'vulnerable children and young people'. This included those with EHCPs who would be expected to attend school where it was appropriate for them, and where there was no requirement for the child to be shielding. Which all sounded like good news as far as we were concerned, although things weren't quite so simple. While two of our boys would fall into this category, they were both at mainstream schools that were now closed. The local authority offered to take them, along with other children in the same situation, at a random school where they'd be taught together like a kind of special needs supergroup – a Traveling Wilburys of local *Zappas* – but this sounded less than ideal, so we passed on the offer. We figured the battle to persuade two teenagers to go to a new school, with new teachers and new peers, would be too great to bother fighting, not least because it would have inevitably cost me a huge amount in bribery. At a time when I wasn't working, this felt like an unnecessary expense.

Anyway, we were less concerned with Adam and Dylan at this point. We had naive visions of them mostly keeping themselves to themselves, doing the occasional lesson on Zoom and then relaxing in front of a screen. Surely, it would take until another pandemic for Dylan to run out of stupid videos to watch on YouTube.* The child we were most concerned about was Zoe. Unlike the boys, she genuinely loves school. She loves her teacher Ian, she loves the classroom assistants, she loves her friends and she's loved all the incarnations of Barry the bus driver. Moreover, she needs the consistency of school and to be kept occupied through the whole day. Given this, we were relieved to read of the government's plans for vulnerable children, and presumed that in Zoe's case she wouldn't even need to go to a different setting. We imagined that since she attends a special school, where every child has an EHCP and so qualifies as 'vulnerable', that it would need to stay open and run almost as normal. Alas, this wasn't the case. The school initially blamed the government's guidance for being confusing, which was understandable to some extent. After all, even Boris Johnson was confused whether he was allowed to host a birthday party during lockdown. More reasonably, the school claimed they didn't have the staff to safely stay open, since many teachers and assistants were shielding.

Even when they eventually reopened, it came with so many caveats that they were practically guaranteed to still have an empty building. Among the provisos was that no pupil could attend if they needed personal care – so that was Zoe and most of her friends done for immediately – and laughably, that 'the pupil has some idea of social distancing'. Considering half the people in our

---

* Spoiler alert: this is not how it turned out.

local Sainsbury's didn't seem to fully comprehend social distancing, what chance was there for a child with Down syndrome? We can't get her to keep her hearing aid on for more than 30 seconds, so I'm not sure we'd have got too far with this one.

The upshot was that Zoe remained at home and became quite depressed during this period. Not in the way I do, of course. She didn't lie in bed listening to the Smiths and reading Sylvia Plath. Nor was she able to tell us how she was feeling, but it was evident that she wasn't herself. She was quieter than normal, wasn't eating as much as she should and was being even more destructive than usual. This book is going to have to shift a lot of units if we want to make good our now ramshackle house.

So, like it or not – and clearly the answer was not – I was forced into home schooling. You might think we'd have been at an advantage here, seeing that Gemma is a teacher who previously worked as a SENDCo and the head of a special school. However, she had her own class to teach, so unfortunately the bulk of the home school-ing fell to me. This wasn't a good thing for anyone, because it's fair to say I'm not the most natural teacher. I decided to base my teaching style on the schoolmasters I had growing up, so I immediately stopped using deodor-ant. It was either that or try to copy my annoying drama teacher who'd say, 'Don't call me Mr Wilkins, call me Steven.' I think every school had one of those. Other teachers would try to intimidate us by showing how clever they were. For example, the head of Junior School, Mr Wilson, would demonstrate his memory by rebuking boys with lines such as:

> You boy!! Stop right there! Ah, I might have known;
> Ashley Blaker, 215 Hartfield Avenue, Elstree, WD6
> 3JJ.

But that method wouldn't have impressed the kids at my home school since their address is also my address. Plus, these are my children we're talking about. I highly doubt any of them even know their own postcode. I think they'd be none the wiser if I gave an Arbroath postcode, such as DD11 1AE.

Having decided on my teaching style, it was time to get to grips with the curriculum. I wanted to provide a balanced timetable that would bring structure to the day. The initial one I came up with looked like this:

9 a.m. – 10 a.m.: Netflix
10 a.m. – 11 a.m.: Amazon Prime
11 a.m. – 12.30 p.m.: Disney+
12.30 p.m. – 1.30 p.m.: Lunch (while watching TikTok)
1.30 p.m. – 2.30 p.m.: Amazon Prime
2.30 p.m. – 3.30 p.m.: Netflix

Unfortunately, I made the stupid mistake of printing this out and sticking it to the wall. I'd forgotten that Gemma would see it and demand I rethink my plans.

As it happens, my children go to Jewish schools and should theoretically spend part of the day studying Judaism and learning Hebrew. I say theoretically, because my children have remarkably little interest in Judaism and are probably less knowledgeable than the average child at Ramallah High. I once asked Dylan, 'What is the holiday that falls around February or March, when we have public celebrations and dress up in funny costumes?' He thought about it for a moment and answered, 'Red Nose Day?'*

Part of my problem during the pandemic was simply having too many children. If you only had one or two kids, at least home school will have provided some precious one-on-one time. However, teaching six of them at once was something else entirely. Not only was I both a teacher and an LSA, I was also simultaneously running a primary school, a secondary school, a special school and a sixth-form college. I wasn't sure whether I should teach them to count, multiplication, quadratic equations or binary logarithms. No educator in the country teaches that range of lessons. It would be like being both a presenter on *Play School* and a lecturer for the Open University.

The sad truth is that much of what I was meant to teach was beyond me. I'm a 40-something whose body is struggling with athlete's foot and haemorrhoids. I can't remember what I had for dinner last night, let alone what I learnt in school in the mid-1980s. I remember something about subsistence farming and the word 'antidisestablishmentarianism', and that's about it. I might be technically what's called highly educated, but none of what I've studied feels relevant to a house full of *Zappas*. My unfinished PhD was entitled 'The doctrine and liturgy of parish clergy removed for Laudianism,

---

* Very well done if you knew the answer is Purim, unless you're Jewish, in which case so what?! You know more than Dylan. That really isn't so impressive!

1641–1642 and their impact on religion in the parishes in the decade before the Long Parliament'. I don't think you'll find the priesthood in the mid-17th century features on the curriculum of many special schools, and definitely not Jewish ones.

I spent most of the time I was meant to be home schooling, looking things up online that I should probably have known already.

What is a rhombus?

What is a compound sentence?

Is a comedian a critical worker whose children should be eligible for key worker school?

In case you're interested, the answers to that last one are no and no, so I couldn't even palm off Edward or The Bailey.

I eventually stopped looking stuff up because I was so paranoid there was some 25-year-old sitting in Google HQ, doubled over with laughter at the things I searched for. I'd rather my children failed their exams than give this millennial hipster the satisfaction of knowing I don't understand the difference between a high-frequency word and a sight word.

With all the kids 'learning' together in our living room, just the noise of everyone on Zoom was enough to drive me mad. Children weren't allowed to attend online lessons in their bedrooms for reasons of child protection, but no one thought about my eardrum protection. And that's before I even got on to dealing with the endless technical issues, which made me feel like I was running a call centre for PC World. I was tempted to affect an Indian accent while insisting my name is really Steve. I wouldn't mind, but my children are so computer literate when it suits them. They were signing themselves up to Snapchat practically the moment they came out the womb. However, when it was a question of accessing online work, they suddenly became less computer savvy than the Handforth Parish Council. My youngest couldn't type in the numbers of a Zoom meeting or unmute herself when required to answer a question, yet last year we discovered she'd set up her own YouTube channel titled 'The Bailey Wants Crisps Now'.

And while I managed to beg, borrow and steal enough computers, inevitably our internet connection was never up to the challenge of allowing five children to participate in online classes. We had so many devices running at once, we'd have needed to move to the Apple Campus in Silicon Valley. Sadly, we're with Virgin Media, which in theory means superfast fibreoptic broadband, but in reality means something closer to CEEFAX in 1985. In lockdown, Wi-Fi became the ultimate commodity in our house, and it was every man, woman and child for themselves. I didn't care if Zoe wanted to stream *Peppa Pig* in Urdu (a change is as good as a rest) or Adam had a pathological need to murder computer-generated street thugs. If it was briefly working, I was racing to get my computer online so I could check if Liverpool had bought any new players. Priorities.

And bravo to any readers who were paying attention and spotted that I said five children having online lessons instead of six. That's because Ollie didn't attend a single class in the entire first lockdown and spent March to September 2020 in his bedroom sleeping. Some of you will be shouting at this point, 'Teenage boys in their room aren't only sleeping!' Well, that's too horrific an image for me to consider, so I'm going with sleeping. But whatever he was doing, it wasn't schoolwork, as barely a day went by when I wasn't sent an email from his teachers complaining about his non-attendance. Thankfully our crap Wi-Fi meant I only had to read them every three or four days. Even worse, Ollie became entirely nocturnal, going to sleep around 9 a.m. When his school finally reopened, he arrived every day just in time to go to bed.

I do feel my children need to shoulder some responsibility for the terrible failure of our home school. To be sure, I exhibited a lack of enthusiasm for home teaching, but this was more than matched by their lack of interest in home learning. It certainly gave me a new appreciation for what their teachers have to put up with, and made me realise that getting Adam or Dylan to engage with their schoolwork is not as easy as I might have imagined. One good thing was that with GCSEs moving to teacher assessment, we at least avoided the trauma of trying to get Adam to revise. He wasn't one of those students whose results were downgraded by algorithm, probably because his predictions were already so low, were he downgraded any further he'd have come out the other side and been top. It's a shame they don't offer GCSEs in *Grand Theft Auto*, Railcard Misplacement or Stealing Phone Chargers. Just as many *Zappas* aren't made for school, they likewise aren't made for exams, and in some ways the pandemic offered a way out from this. Adam still failed them, which was no surprise, but he – and by extension, we – were spared a very stressful experience, which would have been too much for him at that point in his life. By the time he finally had to take proper exams in 2022 he had matured sufficiently that he was able to face them with a degree of calm.

As I write these words, my hope and expectation are that we won't have to go through anything like this again. COVID-19 is still with us, but there's no suggestion that schools will once more close. Furthermore, there was a century between Spanish flu and the coronavirus pandemic, so we should be fine for the rest of our lives.* I'm working on the assumption that all of us can now look back on the lockdowns as a strange and extremely demanding period of our lives. But for us parents of children with SEN it was such an extraordinary trial, I wonder if it will take us quite some time to recover. When our children eventually went back to school, we were demob happy, and that elation probably carried us through the next few months. Yet I think the scars will need a lot longer to heal. So, with that in mind, here are a few things we should remember post-COVID.

1. Go easy on yourself

If you ever feel exhausted and struggle to cope, remember the pandemic. Life was already hard in 2019. Since then we've all been through a lot. Be kind to yourself.

---

* Famous last words, especially as the papers seem to be writing non-stop about monkeypox.

2. Don't take those that support your children for granted

Whether it's their schools, their teachers, their LSAs or other staff. Whether they're amazing, which happily many are, or whether they're completely inept, which applies to some I could name, but which HarperCollins won't let me. Whether they drag you into pointless meetings or whether they're more judicious with your time. During the pandemic we realised how great a role they play in our lives and the lives of our children, and we don't want to be without them again.

3. Watch what you eat

This one is most important. Whatever you do, please, please, please don't eat any food from a Wuhan wet market. Actually, make that any wet market. Or any market. Or anything at all. Just don't eat, don't touch anything, always wear a mask, sanitise your hands and hopefully, God willing, we'll never experience anything like this ever again. I can't speak for you, but I hope I've taught my last lesson of home school.

25

U IS FOR UNBELIEVABLE, BUT THEY REALLY ARE GROWING UP

During this book I've covered the children at various stages of their lives. We've dealt with Adam as the wild three-year-old that a school tried to keep out; Dylan as the eight-year-old who wouldn't stop discussing *The Simpsons* on a flight to Greece; and Zoe as the two-year-old we adopted and then struggled to get dressed in the mornings. To be honest, it's been challenging for me to compute that the little ones I've been writing about are these strapping teenagers I see wandering around my house. Half of them are now taller than me, and at times I've needed to remind myself that they are the same people. They aren't characters in a novel, preserved in aspic in 2008, 2014 or whenever an anecdote was set. Unbelievably, after everything we've been through as a family, they really are growing up.

So what do these children look like as I come to the final chapters? I'd love to say time has healed all and that if you have *Zappas* like mine, all you must do is wait it out; that they've battled through the disabilities and grown out of all their challenging behaviours. It would be a very uplifting way to end the book and no doubt give succour to many readers. Sadly, it wouldn't really be true. Yes, we might be done with nappies and speech therapists, but I sometimes think the real fun is just starting.

Adam is now 18 and has finally left education. After bouncing from school to school, he found his feet at college and, incredibly, having been told he'd never get any qualifications, successfully completed his Level 1 and 2 courses, and managed to pass GCSEs in both English and Maths, albeit at the third attempt.* It's no exaggeration to say that the day he received his results was one of the most joyous in our house. That small boy who could say little more than 'bo' and 'cri' had come a long way, and we were so proud of him. I immediately tweeted the good news and it received thousands of likes, as Twitter users took a brief break from hurling abuse at each other to send their congratulations to Adam. That said, in July 2019 I tweeted:

> A 15-year-old just knocked Venus Williams out at Wimbledon. My eldest son turns 15 tomorrow and he's currently in his bedroom playing Fortnite in his underpants.

This tweet got over 62,000 likes and 7,000 retweets, which I think proves conclusively that people on Twitter would much rather laugh at Adam and humiliate him than celebrate his achievements. Cruel bastards, all of you!

---

* Ever the Jewish mother, Gemma is insisting I point out that in Maths Adam got a 5, so it wasn't as though he only scraped a pass!! Yes, he's practically got an ology.

Adam is a charming, good-looking young man whom, were you to meet for a brief time, you might think was a slightly shy *Coldplay*. A few years ago he'd gained a lot of weight due to a combination of his medication and a preposterously poor diet. However, after being weighed at his annual check-up and told he was in danger of becoming obese, he showed huge will-power to lose over six stone.* He has discovered a love of working out, and is always running or lifting weights. Every time I look at him he's slightly more ripped, and it's hard not to be bowled over by his dedication and discipline.

I'm not sure to what extent Adam's *Coldplay*-like appearance is down to masking – he isn't very forthcoming about his diagnosis and doesn't tend to talk about it – but he has certainly found ways to manage his life as he's matured. He only puts himself in situations in which he's comfortable, and appears to be happy doing his own thing instead of trying to fit in. This should be a good compromise, because I'm aware that masking – the various techniques people use to hide their neurodivergence in certain situations – can be an uncomfortable and exhausting experience.

Yet for those of us that live with Adam his autism is still very much evident, particularly around transitions. As he was about to finish college he became noticeably angrier and even more monosyllabic than usual, which I'm sure was down to his fear of entering the real world. He needs a lot of help with adulting, so when I saw an advert for jobs at McDonald's and suggested he apply, it

---

* Oh, come on Americans, just google it!

led to me spending hours filling in all the forms. At the very least, I'd have liked a free Big Mac for my efforts.

Once Adam gets over his anxieties, he's good humoured and personable. He's been working under the Golden Arches for three months, and he absolutely loves it and seems to be thriving. In fact, the way he walks around the house you'd think he was out there doing deals like Gordon Gekko, the responsibility of the job and extra money in his pocket giving him a new swagger. I don't think it's occurred to him that his minimum-wage salary only appears a lot because his father pays for everything. His ASD means he doesn't like coming face to face with customers at the till, and he still gets nervous about new situations. He told us that he wanted to continue making drinks forever – apparently fries are really hard work – which I feel could be a metaphor for Adam's life as an adolescent with autism. But when forced out of his comfort zone, he can do it. Last week he started on the drive-thru, where he claims, 'Only the toughest survive.' Next stop, *Dragons' Den*.

His diagnosis affects him in other ways that were apparent to me on a recent holiday in New York. He dislikes crowded places and loud noises, so was much happier sitting in a quiet spot in Central Park than going anywhere near Midtown. Yet his sensory needs mean he also likes to be active, and he'd periodically run off for ten minutes, reappearing in a sweat, having done a lap of the block with stops for pull-ups at every bit of scaffolding. His eating is still very limited. During seven days in Manhattan I don't think he ate anything other than chicken burgers. He also lacks the social awareness to avoid situations most people would naturally shy away from. On the subway at night, Adam would engage with those individuals clearly high on meth that everyone else walks down the carriage to avoid. Nor does he notice things that others do. Girls would check him out and smile, but Adam didn't realise at all. He probably came across as aloof, but it's more because he spends much of the time lost in his own world.

I can't say Adam is any more empathetic either. Dylan recently had terrible toothache and was up all night, alternately emitting moans and screams. Adam could hear it, but didn't think to leave his room to find out if he could help. He merely texted Gemma, 'You need to check on Dylan. I think he's watching porn.' The mind boggles as to what Adam has been exposed to if he thinks Dylan's agonising cries are the sounds of sex.

Notwithstanding his decaying teeth, **Dylan** has also grown into a lovely young man who displays his individuality through his long, undercut hair and insistence on only wearing Hawaiian shirts. He looks like a cross between Jay from Kevin Smith's View Askewniverse movies* and Ace Ventura. Unlike Adam, he is very comfortable with his diagnosis, and it's helped him to understand himself and navigate his way through life. In fact, I just asked him how he feels about having autism, and this is what he had to say:

---

* *Clerks, Mallrats, Chasing Amy, Dogma, Jay and Silent Bob Strike Back*, etc.

I fucking love having autism!

It's like having a fast pass for life.

You get to skip lines at theme parks.

It's a brilliant conversation starter.

Girls like autistic boys 'cos it's hot apparently.

People give you sympathy for some reason and I can get away with loads of stuff. At school, half the time I just mention autism and it works. They can't argue back because supposedly it's ableist.

Autism is the best!

Well, I don't condone the swearing, have worries about him using his diagnosis to get away with bad behaviour at school and regret that he's watched so much American TV that he says 'line' instead of 'queue'. But except for those concerns, I'm obviously delighted that he has such a positive attitude towards his autism.

As it happens, he's doing fairly well at school, even though he still has the capacity to surprise his teachers. Last term in English he had to write a book report about John Boyne's Holocaust novel *The Boy in the Striped Pyjamas*. His piece of work ended with the line, 'I rate this book 9.8 out of 10 (didn't have enough comedy).'

Only my gloriously quirky Dylan could read a book about Auschwitz and expect it to include 'a funny thing happened on the way to the gas chambers'.

I also worry about his basic literacy. A few weeks ago he asked if I was free to drop him at a friend's house in Borehamwood. I replied, 'Fine,' and requested the address.

'It's Beef Oven Road,' he informed me.

'What?!'

'Beef Oven Road. She lives at 57 Beef Oven Road.'

'That can't be the address.'

'It is! I promise you. It's Beef Oven Road.'

'Dylan, there's no road in Borehamwood or anywhere in the country called Beef Oven Road.'

Dylan was resolute. 'There is. She texted me the address. Look.' With total certainty, Dylan handed me his phone to see his friend's message on WhatsApp. 'See?'

I took a quick glance. 'Dylan, that's pronounced Beethoven. It's 57 Beethoven Road.'

On second thoughts, this may not be a question of illiteracy and could just reflect his woeful lack of general knowledge. Perhaps he'd simply never heard of the composer and, if this is the case, that's probably a good thing. I'd hate to think he's been going around saying he likes Beef Oven's Symphony No. 5 in C Minor.

As this story indicates, Dylan does have friends, and not just one or two. He's by far the most popular of our children, with a wide social circle and a very close friendship group. Naturally, Gemma and I are overjoyed that he's so well liked, as well as gratified that they all seem nice kids. They appear to get Dylan and appreciate him for who he is, even though what goes on in his brain remains a mystery. He recently went on a ten-day school trip to Italy and was required to take a small amount of stationery. Gemma sent him to the shops with her credit card and he returned an hour later with no pencils or pens but having had a haircut. When she asked why he hadn't bought what he needed, Dylan said he'd forgot, so back he went with strict instructions to go to Ryman's and nowhere else. He came back this time with a Helix maths set, which, while admittedly containing a single pencil, didn't have the other two pencils he required, nor the pens, sharpener or eraser on the list.

Gemma was exasperated. 'Why have you bought this? You don't need a protractor or compass.'

'Yeah, but it was on offer. Look, half price! Such a good deal.'

Dylan may not have been heading to Italy with the right supplies, but at least we knew we were sending him off with the ability to draw a perfect circle.* As Gemma often says, he really shouldn't be let out the house.

Speaking of drawing, Dylan has developed into a hugely gifted artist. He was selected from over a thousand applicants to appear on the BBC series *Britain's Best Young Artist*, and we were thrilled that his talents had been appreciated. Having said this, Dylan felt he didn't do himself justice on the recording, and in many ways this was a result of his diagnosis. The show involved the contestants having to create a work of art against the clock. They were told three weeks in advance what the theme would be and instructed to practise as much as possible so they'd be able to produce something worthy in the allotted time. We were so keen for Dylan to give a good account of himself, we said he didn't need to do any homework and waived all chores – as if he did them anyway – until after the filming. However, Dylan's ADHD being what it is, he couldn't settle down to practise, even with the medication that's meant to help his concentration. Every time we went to his room he was either drawing animation on his iPad or graffitiing the walls in a Banksy-esque style. All brilliant art, but never the one

---

* Plus, we had a spare protractor for when Ollie next loses his.

piece he was meant to be working on. Unsurprisingly, given this, he didn't win his heat, although it was still wonderful to see him on TV when the episode was broadcast and felt like validation of his huge gift.

Unfortunately, his communication skills haven't developed as much as we'd have hoped, considering the countless sessions of speech therapy. He can now speak, to be sure, but he doesn't always understand appropriate interaction, especially when it comes to messaging on his phone. If he misses the bus and wants advice how to get to school, he won't send us a single message and leave it at that. He will send 30 in a row that will look like this.

Dad the bus didn't come so how do I get to school
How
Dad
How
How
Dad
How
Dad
Bus didn't come
How
Dad
How
Dad
How
Dad
Dad
Dad
How
Dad

It is as though his WhatsApp has an echo. Either that or he's very well read and is parodying Molly Bloom's soliloquy in *Ulysses*. I like to occasionally give him a taste of his own medicine and will message again and again about his homework.

> Have you done your history project?
> Have you?
> History
> Project
> History
> Project
> History
> Project
> History
> Project

As they say, if you can't beat 'em, join 'em. Join. 'em. Join. 'em. Join. 'em. Join. 'em.

There are other issues relating to Dylan's autism, not least around empathy. I'm aware this is a thorny issue in the autistic community, with some bloggers arguing that rather than lacking this emotion, they actually have too much of it. Interestingly, I believe Dylan provides evidence for both side of this debate. For example, he doesn't like going to the West End as the sight of homeless people on the street makes him awfully upset. It would be a particularly hard-hearted person who didn't feel sad to see others sleeping rough, but Dylan gets so distressed by their plight that he needs to avoid it altogether. Yet while this suggests he's extremely empathetic, it remains highly selective and, from Gemma's and my perspective, directed towards the wrong places. So, while it's very nice that he feels strongly about the suffering of people he doesn't know, he has absolutely no empathy at all when it comes to The Bailey. Every day he fights with her and always blames his sister:

'Why is she constantly begging for attention?'

'Why does she have so little understanding of the world?'

'Why does she believe all the bullshit she watches on YouTube?'

If you can overlook for a moment the unbelievable *chutzpah* of Dylan accusing anyone of taking their opinions from YouTube, what's apparent is that he lacks the sensitivity to appreciate a key point: that The Bailey is eight years old! That's why she doesn't know much about the world, why she can't tie her own shoelaces and why she sings songs from *The Greatest Showman* morning, noon and night. It's nothing to do with her being 'stupid' – which should itself be a reason to have sympathy – but simply a function of being seven years his junior.

Last month The Bailey was crying because Dylan had called her 'a fucking bitch'. I told him he'd be losing his pocket money, and Dylan was furious and genuinely couldn't see what he'd done wrong. Not only did he feel it was perfectly justified – The Bailey had apparently said she was pescatarian even though she eats Chicken McNuggets – he also wanted to argue semantics with me. According to Dylan he hadn't called her a fucking bitch: he'd said she was 'acting like a fucking bitch'. He was adamant that saying a person is acting like something is completely different to saying they are literally that thing. In the end I gave him his pocket money back just to shut him up and we all tried to move on from 'Fuckingbitchgate'.

While in some regards – and only some! – Adam and Dylan have got easier as they've matured, **Zoe** has unquestionably become harder. We now have a hormonal teenager with the mental age of a four-year-old, but unlike a four-year-old she's not in bed by half-six. She's too heavy to carry upstairs when she refuses to have a bath; too contrary to eat dinner when it's served; too frightened of dogs to go outside; and too bored to sit in the house for more than half an hour. She's watched every episode of *Peppa Pig* in Gujarati, and I've so far failed to get her into *Charlie and Lola* in Cantonese.

Like a toddler, she'll cry in the night and wake everyone if her duvet has moved just five centimetres out of position. But in other ways she resembles a teenager. I assume Zoe's recently started some form of sex ed in school, because she repeatedly says to Gemma, 'I was in your tummy.' Not a spoiler by this point: she wasn't. I'm convinced she's even started using sign language insolently, but my Google searches for 'bolshy Makaton' have yet to yield any results. She really needs dedicated one-to-one care, which is why she loves her residential camp in the summer and Christmas holidays. What can I say? No one asked us to adopt her!

I know many people in the autistic community hate the portrayal of autism in *Rain Man* and the like, but I've an even greater problem with the representation of those with Down syndrome in the media, albeit for the opposite reason. Barely a week goes by that I don't see articles about amazing individuals with DS who've achieved all manner of things: presenting an award at the Oscars;

modelling for Victoria's Secret; running a highly successful cookie business. The implication is that Down
syndrome shouldn't be a hindrance, but in Zoe's case it
most certainly is. Don't get me wrong. It's wonderful that
these stories are out there and I'm delighted that these
incredible people are changing perceptions. However,
they make me question if we've somehow failed as
parents when an achievement for our 14-year-old daughter isn't winning a BAFTA but not vandalising the house
beyond repair.

Many is the time we've taken our eye off Zoe and
found her stuffing wet wipes down the toilet, emptying
salt onto the kitchen counter, cutting her hair off with
nail scissors or using felt-tip pens to graffiti the walls, or
more often her clothes and face. On the positive, her
make-up is much cheaper than her sister's. The Bailey
wants Elizabeth Arden or Estée Lauder; Zoe is perfectly
happy with Crayola. The negative is that the saving
doesn't cover the cost of the plumber, who's a frequent
visitor to our house to unblock the toilet. I've thought
about pinching more pennies by downgrading her to
Poundland's own-brand pens, but the financial benefit
would be negligible. Even worse, there have been times
she's drawn on herself with semi-permanent markers,
and we've had to send her to school with a note asking to
forgive the fact she now looks like the rapper Post Malone.

Occasionally we try to entertain her by arranging playdates with friends from her class, but these are usually
more trouble than they're worth, as demonstrated by a
recent meet-up with Benji. Zoe was extremely excited
and talked about nothing else all week.

'Benji today?' she'd ask every morning of the holidays.

'No, Zoe. Benji on Thursday,' we'd explain to much disappointment.

On the morning of the playdate she was beside herself. This was the most animated she'd been since coming back from camp. Yet when they finally met at a local park – not a great idea to take Zoe to where there are so many dogs, but still better than letting Benji loose in our house – they ignored each other and played almost entirely separately. Their sole interaction was taking it in turns to periodically wander over to the other.

'I hate you.'

'No, I hate you.'

Then they'd head off in opposite directions before returning to profess their mutual hatred a few minutes later.

Despite all of this, Zoe remains a light in our life, and a kiss and a cuddle from her is enough to make me forget the many challenges. She may be a teenager, but there's still a remarkable innocence about her. Every day The Bailey finds new cosmetics, clothes or cuddly toys that she simply must have or she's going to die, while Zoe has literally never asked us to buy her anything, even though she's bombarded with adverts on YouTube. They simply bounce off her as if she were Supergirl. She doesn't have a phone, isn't on TikTok, never stays up all night chatting with friends, hasn't become obsessed with her weight and wouldn't know Harry Styles if he sat down at our kitchen table, let alone make me take her to see him in concert. For that alone I'll love Zoe forever (apologies, Harries). And while she might never run a business or star in a BBC drama, we didn't adopt her with any thought that these would be possible. People often ask me why we did it and I always echo the mountaineer George Mallory. Because she was there. Do I wish it were easier? Of course, but this is who we took on. And now I think about it, she performed as herself in my Radio 4 series, so she's appeared in a world-renowned show after all.

That's where our *Zappas* are at. And what of the children still technically considered *Coldplays*?

Ollie is about to start his A-levels, having achieved an impressive mix of 7s, 8s and 9s in his GCSEs. He has thankfully passed through the stinky teen phase and looks very smart in his new clothes for sixth form. I did worry, because for a time he didn't seem fussed about trivial things like washing or using deodorant. He worked throughout the pandemic in a busy local supermarket and never got ill, which I think suggests his personal hygiene was so bad that not only did everyone wear a mask and stay two metres away, but COVID itself didn't want to be inside his stinky body. Although thank God for small mercies, because the one thing worse than teenagers who smell of B.O. is teenagers who smell of body spray. I think I prefer the stench of our family bathroom to Lynx Africa.*

I still have my doubts over whether Ollie is a definite *Coldplay*. When I took him to buy his new wardrobe for school, he became stressed because we bought one jumper from Next and another from Uniqlo. He was insistent that both his jumpers must be from the same

---

* Little-known fact: Lynx is secretly bankrolled by American Christian groups, being as it is the most effective way to prevent teenagers having sex.

shop. I didn't probe him on why because after years of dealing with Adam and Dylan's demands about clothing, I can't cope with much more. Perhaps all the years in Adam's company have influenced him. Yes, that must be it. I am not willing to entertain any other possibility at this stage. What I do know is that Ollie is a very intelligent young man with a bright future ahead of him.

As he approaches his teens, **Edward** is for the time being still a sweet, good-natured little boy, even though he strikes me as more autistic than Adam and Dylan combined. His hyperfixations are only intensifying; he'd rather google 'brilliant goats' than spend time with friends; and his dubious social skills lead him to have frequent disagreements with other children over WhatsApp, which nearly always end with him going nuclear and blocking them. Literally five minutes ago he insisted I forward him an email from UPS saying they have his LEGO set. He wants to stare at it. There's much about Edward that's hard to explain. Two days ago, on a trip to a shopping centre, he walked around shouting the names of dinosaurs. Quite why he felt the need to loudly proclaim '*Spinosaurus!*' and '*Diplodocus!*' is anyone's guess, and I don't feel adequately qualified to give an answer. Still, he's only 12 and, if Adam's anything to go by, a lot will change in the next few years. For now I'm just grateful that I still have one boy who likes cuddling me on the sofa and I'll enjoy it while it lasts.

As for **The Bailey**, at eight years of age she has even more maturing to do, although in many ways she's already grown up far too fast. On our recent summer holiday Gemma asked her to change out of the dress she'd worn two days running. Immediately The Bailey shot back, 'My body, my choice.' Gemma was stumped. How could she answer and somehow not undermine her own feminist principles and commitment to bodily autonomy? Anyway, The Bailey had already spoken so much on the plane that by this point Gemma was all talked out and had little left to give. Not even Johnny Vine ever experienced anything to compare with eight hours of listening to The Bailey. Had Amnesty International heard about it, they'd have reported her to the UN for violation of Gemma's human rights.

And yet, while we might find The Bailey a challenge, her extrovert personality charms other people. She's been blessed with a natural aptitude for making relationships and drawing people to her in a way I've never experienced with our *Zappas*. She makes friends with other children both at school and in public places; she chats with checkout staff; and her inherent charisma is such that she managed to schmooze a fierce-looking immigration officer at JFK Airport and get us moved to the front of the queue for passport control. All of this suggests her pathway through life will be easier than for my boys, and means I have less cause for concern about her future.

To keep face-to-face interaction with the children to a bare minimum, we now have a Blaker family WhatsApp group, comprising me, Gemma and the four boys.* Primarily, the group is used for Gemma to post complaints about the children, usually for not cleaning

---

* Zoe doesn't have a phone and wouldn't be mentally capable of taking part anyway. Meanwhile, The Bailey asks for her own phone at least three times a day, but we're making her wait until she's in Year 6.

up after themselves in the kitchen. It's great that the big boys have become more independent and will now cook their own meals after we've gone to bed. It's just a shame this involves using every single utensil, which they never wash up, creating a trail of pasta all over the floor and leaving open each cupboard door for good measure. It's both dispiriting and slightly comical to wake in the morning to Gemma's venting in the group. In the last month alone she's posted this selection that I think says everything you need to know about living with my teenage boys:

> The mess in the bathroom is ridiculous! If you take new toothpaste, throw the old one away. Shut the drawer. And put the package in the bin. Whoever did this needs to sort it out and pick the towels off the floor.

> If you are taking a drink, you don't need to take three different mugs that I have to wash up. Use the same mug all evening please.

> Who has taken Bailey's donuts out of the utility room? I went to Sainsbury's especially to get them this morning.

> I have organised the sauces in the cupboard. Please don't buy anything until you've checked what we've got. We don't need seven bottles of sweet chilli sauce!

OK I've cleaned the mess that Zoe made with the shampoo in the bath. It took ages so if you are washing your hair in the bath, please put the shampoo and conditioner on the side so she can't reach them.

Someone last night has done the most enormous disgusting poo all over the downstairs toilet. You are now old enough to clean this up yourself and not leave it for me when it is dried in and impossible to remove. If that happens take a cloth and some spray and clean it!!! I am not the family slave!

My all-time favourite, however, was:

Remember that the electrician is coming tomorrow at 12. PLEASE be polite and not make him think we're nuts.

Adam replied that the electrician mustn't disturb him, because he needs to be able to rest now that he's working. Fair enough, he has to be fresh and on top of his game if he's going to make the perfect McFlurry.

Of course, the WhatsApp group is open to abuse, which usually involves Dylan. When he went on his recent school trip to Italy, he was posting furiously from the bus to the airport:

What's our Netflix login?
Can anyone help?
Please?

Anyone know the Netflix login?
Help
Help
Help
And anyone know the Disney+
Help
Netflix
Disney+
Netflix
Disney+
Please

It didn't occur to him to ask in advance. Instead, he waited until 5 a.m. on the morning of the flight, when everyone except Gemma would be fast asleep.

Our children seem to revel in making our lives as difficult as possible. Literally yesterday, Gemma announced via the group that on the upcoming bank holiday Monday, she'd be driving down to the beach. We're past the stage of loading everyone into the car and taking them out for the day. Now, we put it out there and the kids can opt in if they wish. If they want to come, then great; if they'd rather stay at home lying in their fetid sheets or watching *Jurassic World Dominion* for the 15th time, that's fine too. Aren't we good parents allowing our children to make their own decisions! Well, if we are, it's never rewarded with anything but acrimony and the kind of complex negotiations that make Brexit seem easy.

Within minutes of Gemma's post, the replies started arriving. Surprisingly, Adam wanted to come, but only on condition Zoe didn't. On being informed that Zoe was joining, Adam said he'd stay at home, which meant now Ollie changed his mind because his attendance was provisional on whether Adam would be there. Dylan said he'd come if he got to sit in the front, and when told he'd be in the back, replied he'd only sit next to Bailey if he was rewarded with three takeaways. Gemma probably thought she'd negotiated well by haggling Dylan down to one, but on seeing this, Adam decided he'd come after all, so he could likewise claim a free chicken burger. This brought Ollie back into the picture, but merely until Adam remembered that he'd be working on Monday, so he was out, as was Ollie. Meanwhile, Edward had initially wanted to stay at home – *Jurassic World Dominion* won't watch itself, and apparently gets better after the 14th viewing – but, on realising Ollie would be in the house, and therefore pulling rank to use the TV, announced that he wanted to attend. However, Edward requested that he be allowed to bring his school friend, Obsessed-with-Warhammer Brown. This led to Dylan asking to be accompanied by No-Way-He'll-Ever-Hold-Down-a-Job Turner or Too-Fucked-Up-for-Words Simmonds. There are still three days to go, and your guess is as good as mine as to who will end up in the car to the beach.

So that's my children as they are today. They are no longer the little ones responsible for 'Butchergate', 'Policegate' and 'Foamgate', but they are still wonderfully disobedient, irreverent and determined to do their own thing. Most importantly, I love them all very much, even though they often make it as hard as possible to do so. Normal schmormal! I wouldn't have them any other way.

26

O IS FOR ONWARDS AND UPWARDS

A few years ago, amid typically chaotic scenes around the kitchen table, Ollie looked at me and Gemma, and with a straight face asked a couple of difficult questions.

'Why is everyone in this house so weird? Why can't our family just be normal?'

Most things that get said in our home I take with a pinch of salt, but this was different. This really hurt since I knew it was true. We aren't 'normal', and I'd have hoped that Ollie could enjoy this fact and, rather than wishing it away, appreciate having such gloriously idiosyncratic siblings.

That's also my wish for you. That if your children are in any way like mine, that you and everyone in your lives values them for who they are, instead of craving normality, whatever that is. Of course, this is easier said than done, and it's taken us quite some time to reach this place of acceptance. So, to conclude this book, here are some final suggestions on how to come to terms with raising *Zappas* of any description.

1. Success doesn't always look the same

This is so hard to remember, but it couldn't be more important. Achievement has many faces. When I tweeted about Adam passing his GCSEs, numerous parents replied with stories of their own children's success: people with autism who'd variously received top grades in their A-levels, obtained first-class degrees or been hired for impressive sounding jobs. (Thanks everyone for making Adam's exam results seem less special!) But the tweet that really caught my eye was this one:

> Our six-year-old son has autism and today we
> managed a successful trip to the barbers. It's these
> little things others never have to worry about, that
> when they go well it's a relief.

Yes! This is what I believe they call a hard relate. Mums and dads of *Coldplays* would never dream of considering an incident-free haircut as any kind of triumph, but us parents of *Zappas* have a different reality. For years my boys refused to go to the hairdresser, and I had to do it – badly I might add! – while they wore an Iron Man mask from Adam's dress-up, which they believed would stop hair getting in their mouths. In case you wondered, it didn't work, and nor did a rubber Incredible Hulk mask.

For my part I'm going to try to remember the exact same message when it comes to this book. Success doesn't necessarily mean selling millions of copies and getting great reviews. If just one person reading this book feels ... oh, who am I kidding? Success would be selling millions of copies. Damn my fucking ego!

2. Let go of your dreams

We all have visions of what our children will look like. Usually this involves them being miniaturised clones, combining our best qualities and interests with the ability to avoid our mistakes, not that I would ever admit to having made any. But this is illusory. The real task of parenting is to make peace with what you've been given; to offer unconditional love and support without trying to them turn it into something they're not; and then to celebrate them and enjoy it all as much as you can.

It can be tough to accept that our idealised family life is never going to happen. I once suggested a day trip to the Battle of Britain Air Show, which, as I explained to the kids, included flying displays of vintage aircraft. I added dramatic emphasis to my voice when I mentioned the 'staged airfield attack scenario', which I hoped would make it sound more appealing, even though I had no clue what this was. My voiceover skills clearly weren't up to scratch because Adam wasn't impressed.

'What a load of total fucking shit,' my then 14-year-old said. 'No way am I going to that. You'd have to kill me first.'

The Battle of Britain Air Show is exactly the kind of thing my imagined family would have done on a Sunday afternoon. They'd have booked tickets, driven to Duxford, played games in the car on the way there, enjoyed a picnic, and created memories while having fun and learning at the same time. Instead, the day of the air show we spent gathered on the sofa watching videos of cats on treadmills, followed by sharing a party bucket from KFC. And everyone was happy, because we gave them the experience they wanted rather than the idyllic childhood of my dreams.

Unless you want to live in a hell of should-haves and might-have-beens, I suggest that you start giving your *Zappas* what they ask for, rather than what you think they need. (The same goes for your *Coldplays* too, if they don't look like your fantasy mini-me.) It will save a lot of mental anguish and may even bring some joy and connection, especially if you like fried chicken.

3. Try parenting less

Writing this book has obviously offered me a chance to reflect and think how we've done as parents. I realise that sounds very depressing. But while I'm sure many readers will think we've done a terrible job, the conclusion I've come to is that our biggest problem's not that our parenting is bad, but rather that it's just too good!

Yes, you read that right, it wasn't a whole series of typos. Let me explain. We've spent years doing everything for our children. We're not so much carers as glorified PAs, if PAs spent most their time cleaning up your mess, and listening to you drone on and on about dinosaurs. It's no wonder the kids spend all their time endlessly watching inappropriate YouTube videos while fighting over crisps and phone chargers, because Gemma and I have been doing everything else for them.

Of course, some of the children do need serious help. There are many things that Zoe can't do for herself and probably never will. But I've discovered that the others are perfectly capable of looking after themselves when required. A few years ago I noticed Adam was wearing a new belt that we had no recollection of buying him. We enquired and it turned out he had envied Odd-as-Fuck Levy's cool new belt, so he gathered his pocket money, went to the shops on his own, and bought one for himself. He even took it to the dry cleaner for them to punch new holes into it so it would fit perfectly. This is a boy who wouldn't have washed his hands after using the toilet had I not stood there dispensing the soap.* But what 'Beltgate' showed me was that when the motivation was there, our children could be autonomous after all.

More recently, Gemma and I returned home from Starbucks to discover the kids had independently combated the huge number of summer flies in our house by all sitting quietly with white pillowcases over their heads. And OK, it was rather odd to see my children resembling a junior division of the Ku Klux Klan. But they were using their own resourcefulness because their fear of flies was sufficiently important to them to do something about it. Personally, I'd have gone for fly spray ahead of adopting the white supremacist look, and Gemma was none too pleased that our pillowcases now had little holes cut out of them. However, the key point is that without us around they were willing to do some-

---

* Don't worry McDonald's customers, he's improved on that front now!

thing for themselves. Hence my suggestion to you is go start that series on Netflix you keep meaning to watch and stop trying to parent so hard. All that's required is to be there when they need you and offer guidance in the full knowledge that it will be ignored.

4. Sometimes you need to ignore the tears

When Zoe came to live with us in March 2011 she spent the first month crying. She'd been happy and settled with her foster family, and now she'd been wrenched away and forced to cohabit with a bunch of noisy and socially awkward strangers. I can't blame her: there are times I too cry because I have to share a house with her brothers. It was awful, though, and Gemma and I were wracked with guilt. We briefly felt like child abductors and genuinely wondered if we'd done something wrong.

Yet we soon came to our senses and were able to recognise that while this was an incredibly painful experience for Zoe, it was in her best interest in the long run. Her lack of understanding meant she couldn't appreciate this, but she was slowly forging a bond with her forever family that will hopefully never be broken. As formative as that time may have been, I'm sure Zoe now has no memory of ever living with Laura and Ian, and she's very happy with us, at least when the Wi-Fi is working and her iPad hasn't run out of charge.

There have been several moments over the past 12 years when I've reminded myself of this period, because it's such a powerful parable for parenting all our kids, especially the *Zappas*. When you have children with limited understanding, it's often necessary to make decisions for them. They might not like them and might cry their eyes out, but you must trust your better judgement and not let yourself be influenced by the tears. Dylan was devastated when we changed his school in the middle of Year 4. He lay in bed sobbing uncontrollably, mourning his separation from the same classmates he'd complained every day for three months had been bullying him. I'm not sure we've got every call right, but we're the adults and back ourselves to see the bigger picture, even if it causes some short-term weeping.

5. Learn your triggers

Being a parent to *Zappas* can be overwhelming and highly triggering, be it overhearing other parents in the playground, fraught meetings with your child's school, countless hospital appointments, unruly playdates or just idiots talking unsolicited shit to you about your child. But whatever situation it is that gets to you most, I have one overriding piece of advice. Know yourself! Acknowledge which circumstances are your biggest triggers and avoid them like the plague. I'm tempted at this point to tell you mine, but I worry that someone who dislikes me will buy this book simply to hate-read it and will engineer it for me to face my most traumatic scenarios. Actually, do you know what I find most triggering? When people send me cash via the publisher. I really hate that and would do anything to avoid it!*

6. Remember, it's a marathon not a sprint

As it happens I loathe that phrase. It's so trite and often not even true. Someone once said it to Usain Bolt just before he ran the 100m at the Olympics and he ended up last.† But in our particular case I can see it's correct, because after all the shit we've been through we have children who I believe are maturing into wonderful young people. Now this doesn't mean your *Zappa*, who currently doesn't speak and can't attend mainstream school, will definitely end up passing his GCSEs. Who knows what the future holds, but I do know that what happens when they're little isn't the be-all and end-all.

We suffered years of parents' evenings where teachers told us our children seem to feel the normal rules don't apply to them. But as embarrassing as this was, I remain convinced that in the long run this tendency, along with several other of their character traits, will serve them well. When they were younger, Adam and Dylan lived in a glorious bubble of self-certainty, and I hope they can retain that as adults. For now, we have an

---

* Oh, if you insist, then. My biggest trigger is seeing the phone number of any of my children's schools flash up on my phone. It's never going to be good news. Thankfully, I don't think Ronald McDonald knows my number, so at least I'm in the clear when it comes to Adam.

† To be clear, I made that story up.

18-year-old who thinks nothing of talking about Pornhub one minute and watching episodes of *Scooby-Doo* the next. We have a 14-year-old who has an art installation in his bedroom called 'The Nut Room'. Contrary to its name, this is nothing to do with masturbation but is, according to Dylan, a 'mancave dedicated to a belief, with a carpet, a chair and a wall of fame, and is intended as an abstract art design of nut solidity'. So now you know.* Then we have another son who, when I asked if he understood his trigonometry homework, replied, 'Some things we just aren't meant to know.' How wonderful if in the future they could still be this comfortable in their own skin, and not feel ashamed if they seem different or weird.

I'd like to think I've always been someone content to find my own way, but our kids do this very unconsciously, and for this I am proud of them. Sadly, our education system isn't geared to nurturing children who don't easily fit in. But I'm confident there will be a time when my children's unique talents will shine because, well, it's a marathon, not a sprint. And I'd like to add it's a Marathon, not a Snickers, because I can do all that Peter Kay 'Do you remember Spangles?' stuff too.

Their teachers might not be impressed, but I'm delighted that we have such interesting, distinctive children who don't boringly adhere to normal societal expectations. So maybe this means Gemma and I are doing a really great job, raising kids who in all their anarchic, non-conformist glory are going to one day become

---

* If you missed it, head back to 'E is for Embarrassing Photos' for a picture of Dylan in The Nut Room.

truly amazing adults. It's just a shame it also means they make pretty crap children.

7. Sincerely believe in diversity

We live in a world that supposedly champions diversity. We are used to turning on the TV and seeing people of colour, openly gay performers, comedians with cerebral palsy, transgender presenters and occasionally even Northerners. However, most people don't really practise what they preach and they find it hard to take the message on board. We might be happy to see diverse faces in the media – unless we're dickheads, in which case we're not – but we're often unwilling to accept that our friends and family can be different to us. Most people mix only with carbon copies of themselves and avoid anyone that isn't the same.

As parents of *Zappas*, one thing Gemma and I have needed to do is truly embrace diversity. We've had to accept that our children's reality is totally different to ours. They don't think like us and they don't act like us, and that's fine. When I order something from Amazon, I don't lovingly stare at the confirmation email and then track the UPS delivery man like a bona fide stalker. But I know a boy who does, and that's OK because that's his way of doing things. The last time a LEGO set didn't arrive on the day Edward had expected, he was inconsolable. I told Adam to cheer him up, so he walked straight to Edward's bedroom, opened the door and said, 'Don't be such a fucking baby,' before walking off again. For Adam, that's *his* way of doing things. And in a properly diverse world, all approaches are fair and should be respected.

8. Stop looking for answers

There's a great scene at the end of the original *Planet of the Apes* movie, just before Charlton Heston discovers the remains of the Statue of Liberty.* He has the orangutan leader Dr Zaius tied up on the beach and says there must be an answer as to why apes have evolved from man. Zaius replies prophetically, 'Don't look for it, Taylor. You may not like what you find.'

We all crave answers, and having *Zappas* only amplifies the urge. You might want to read books, do research and harvest opinions in the hope they'll provide that elusive magic cure. But as useful as some of these works are – and clearly, the book you hold in your hand is amazing and one that you'll post about all over social media – sometimes it's best to just not know. I'm certainly not advocating that parents don't educate themselves. But guides can only tell you so much. Every child is unique, even if they have the same diagnosis. I have two boys with autism – ahem, two boys *diagnosed* with autism – and they are completely different. One is the shy boy who manages his autism by staying mostly at home; the other is the popular child with the large group of friends whose addresses he can't read. Only you know your child, so trust your instinct and listen to your

---

* Apologies for the spoiler. But if you've not seen it by now, I'm guessing you weren't ever going to get round to it.

wisdom. I did say right at the start that this isn't an outright guidebook, and while it might be an A–Z, it isn't even in the right order. That's because there's no roadmap. You need to find your own way.

9. The future is bright

Well, I hope it is anyway, and that's my sincere blessing to you, my dear reader. I would never have believed that the wild little boy from *D is for Diagnosis Autism* could get GCSEs in English and Maths. He's not perfect but then, to use another well-worn aphorism, 'perfect is the enemy of good'; a phrase I've repeated several times to my editor during the writing of this book. I'd never have believed that the little girl who cried for a month when we adopted her would one day feel so at home with her new family. And I'd never have believed that Dylan would not only talk, but be able to do so on national TV and not make a total twat of himself. There's always optimism for the future.

I hope you've enjoyed our time together. We must do this again some time. Maybe we can meet up in the park and let our kids chase each other while screaming and swearing. (Please don't bring any dogs!) We can sit on a bench, watch the chaos unfold as all the parents of *Coldplays* scarper in terror, and celebrate our magnificently special children. Normal schmormal; typical schmypical; conformity schmonformity; expectations schmexpectations. You get what I'm saying.